# PSYCHOPHYSIOLOGICAL RECORDING

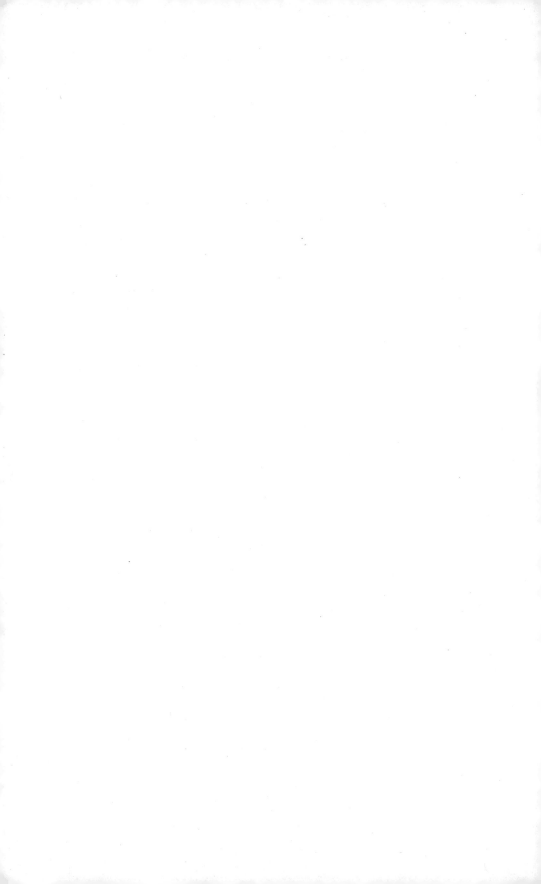

# PSYCHOPHYSIOLOGICAL RECORDING

*Second Edition*

Robert M. Stern
William J. Ray
Karen S. Quigley

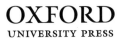
UNIVERSITY PRESS

2001

# OXFORD

UNIVERSITY PRESS

Oxford   New York
Athens   Auckland   Bangkok   Bogotá   Buenos Aires   Calcutta
Cape Town   Chennai   Dar es Salaam   Delhi   Florence   Hong Kong   Istanbul
Karachi   Kuala Lumpur   Madrid   Melbourne   Mexico City   Mumbai
Nairobi   Paris   São Paulo   Shanghai   Singapore   Taipei   Tokyo   Toronto   Warsaw

and associated companies in
Berlin   Ibadan

Copyright © 2001 by Oxford University Press, Inc.

Published by Oxford University Press, Inc.
198 Madison Avenue, New York, New York 10016

Oxford is a registered trademark of Oxford University Press.

Library of Congress Cataloging-in-Publication Data
Stern, Robert Morris, 1937–
Psychophysiological recording / Robert M. Stern, William J. Ray, Karen S. Quigley.—2nd ed.
p. cm.
ISBN 0-19-511358-6; ISBN 0-19-511359-4 (pbk)
1. Psychophysiology—Research—Methodology   I. Ray, William J., 1945–   II. Quigley, Karen S.
QP360 .S79   2000
612.8'028'7—dc21      99-049560

9  8  7  6  5  4  3  2

Printed in the United States of America
on acid-free paper

Dedicated to
R. C. Davis
(1902–1961)
*Teacher, Scholar, and Father*

# Preface

This second edition of our book was written 20 years after the first. There have been great technological advances made during this period, advances that now make possible the recording of additional physiological measures from brain and periphery under a variety of conditions not thought possible when we wrote the first edition. Consider the fact that functional magnetic resonance imaging (fMRI) is now being used in several laboratories to monitor changes in blood flow in the brain, and on a recent NASA mission the electrogastrogram (EGG) was used to measure gastric myoelectric activity from a freely moving astronaut in zero gravity.

We have seen a considerable increase in interest in psychophysiology during the past 20 years, partly due to the availability of new recording techniques, and, we believe, partly due to the birth and enormous growth in the area of cognitive neuroscience. Just as psychophysiology (even before it was called that) contributed both recording techniques and new hypotheses to the study of emotions, it is now making equally valuable contributions to the study of cognition.

This second edition of our book, like the first, was written for those who wish to begin studying psychophysiology. We assumed no previous knowledge of psychophysiology or of related areas such as physiology or instrumentation. Therefore, chapters dealing with these areas are presented first. We aim to provide the reader with a good foundation to begin working in, as well as understanding, psychophysiology.

Every chapter has been updated, and a chapter dealing with signal processing has been added. The book is organized into three parts. Part I deals with background material that we feel is essential to an understanding of psychophysiology. It concludes with a chapter on safety and ethics. Part II presents separate chapters on the psychophysiology of the brain, muscles, eyes, respiratory system, gastrointestinal system, cardiovascular system, skin, and signal processing. Part III deals with applications of psychophysiological recording to research and clinical use.

In addition to serving as the primary text for a course in psychophysiology, this book can function as a supplementary text for courses in biological psychology, neuropsychology, behavioral neuroscience, cognitive neuroscience, human physiology, medical and nursing courses that deal with the recording of physiological measures, and beginning courses in biomedical engineering.

The authors thank our students and others who have commented on the first edition of the book. We also thank the following individuals who have helped with the preparation of this second edition. Kari Logel was a super assistant to the authors. Peter J. Gianaros contributed material to chapter 5, and he read and offered constructive comments on the entire manuscript. Kenneth R. Jones, at the University of North Carolina, also read the entire manuscript and made many valuable suggestions. We are also grateful to Richard G. Lyons of Sunny Vale, California, who contributed his signal processing expertise to our new chapter 14. It is also our pleasure to acknowledge the help, encouragement, and patience of our editor at Oxford University Press, Joan Bossert, and her assistant Constanza Morales-Mair.

# Contents

## PART III. APPLICATIONS

## PART I

# General Elements of Psychophysiology

# 1

## Psychophysiology

Psychophysiology is relatively new as a separate discipline; in the mid-1950s a group of physiological psychologists began referring to themselves as psychophysiologists. However, the subject matter of psychophysiology—the interaction of mind and body—has been studied for centuries by people trained as philosophers, physicists, physicians, physiologists, and, most recently, psychologists.

John Stern (1964) defined the work of psychophysiology as "any research in which the dependent variable (the subject's response) is a physiological measure and the independent variable (the factor manipulated by the experimenter) a behavioral one." If subjects are shown slides, some of landscapes and some of car accident scenes, and the subjects' heart rates are recorded, we have an example of a psychophysiological experiment according to Stern's definition. The dependent variable is heart rate and the independent variable is type of slide (landscape or car accident scene). This study would exemplify the typical psychophysiological experiment in which something was done to the subject and the subject's physiological responses were recorded. Rather than viewing slides, the subject might have been solving problems, experiencing an embarrassing situation, waiting to receive an electric shock, or watching a radar screen for signs of enemy planes. Rather than heart rate, the physiological response recorded might have been sweating; a change in blood pressure, muscle potentials, or cortisol levels in saliva; change in the size of the pupil of the eye; alterations in brain waves, respiration, stomach motility, or penis size; or any of several other bodily changes.

Stern's definition of psychophysiology is not incorrect, but with the passage of time it has become too limiting. The type of research he was defining, as just described, examined the physiological changes that accompanied certain psychological or behavioral manipulations. More recent experiments conducted by psychophysiologists show that it is equally tenable to manipulate physiological variables and examine behavioral changes. In a study typical of newer research, the heart rate of subjects was modified by *biofeedback* and their ability to withstand pain measured. (A glossary is provided at the back of the book that includes definitions of technical terms. These terms are italicized the first time they appear in the text.) The dependent variable in this case is a behavioral one: the indication of how much pain the subject can tolerate. The independent variable is a physiological one: the subject's heart rate.

Psychophysiologists are not the only group of behavioral scientists who study the relationship of physiological and psychological variables. Psychophysiologists are a subset of a larger group of behavioral scientists who were referred to as physiological psychologists until recently, and are now referred to as biological psychologists, psychobiologists, or behavioral neuroscientists. What are some of the differences in the approaches used by psychophysiologists and these other types of biological psychologists? Other biological psychologists usually study the effects of their manipulation of the brain or other parts of the nervous system on some aspect of behavior. The independent variable might be destruction of a part of the brain, while the dependent variable might be eating behavior. Such research must be conducted on nonhuman animals and only rarely on human beings. Most psychophysiologists, on the other hand, study the responses of humans rather than nonhuman animals; therefore, such researchers must limit their techniques of data collection to the surface recording of bioelectric signals. Harmless electrodes are attached to the skin over the organ of interest. The techniques of psychophysiology have the advantage of not greatly interfering with normal behavior, particularly when some of the newer methods (such as ambulatory assessment) are used so that the subjects can move freely (Fahrenberg & Myrtek, 1996). Conversely, because surface recording is used, for example, from the scalp (rather than from deep in the brain), psychophysiologists must sacrifice some degree of immediate biological exactitude, that is, they cannot gain access to the precise source of the bioelectric signal. A biological psychologist might drill a hole through the bony skull of the subject, perhaps a cat, and place a very small electrode on a single cell in a precise part of the brain. This researcher could then record the electrical signal from this cell while studying, for example, pleasure. The psychophysiologist placing electrodes on the surface of the scalp must record the activity of perhaps millions of cells and cannot say much about the nature of the cells, their number, their location, and so on. But the psychophysiologist usually records from human subjects. So when studying pleasure, such a researcher can simply ask subjects to describe how they feel, rather than needing to make assumptions about their feeling state based on observable behavior, as biological psychologists must do. And if the biological psychologist discovers some relationship between the subjects' brain activity and their behavior, this type of researcher still must question whether that same relationship would be found with human subjects. Neither approach, that of psychophysiologists or that of other biological psychologists, is better than the other. They have both contributed and will continue to contribute to our overall understanding of the relationship of physiological and psychological variables.

## Short History and Long Past

The history of psychophysiology as a separate discipline is quite brief. The formal development of psychophysiology began in the 1950s, when a group composed mainly of psychologists met informally under the leadership of R. C. Davis. In 1960 this group organized the Society for Psychophysiological Research, with Chester Darrow as the first president. Research communications among this group were initiated in 1955, when Albert Ax began a newsletter dealing with research and instrumentation in psychophysiology. In 1964 this newsletter developed into the journal *Psychophysiology*, with Ax as the editor; this journal became the society's official publication. Two articles in the first issue of *Psychophysiology* are of historical interest: "Psychophysiology, Yesterday, Today, and Tomorrow" by Darrow (1964), and "Goals and Methods of Psychophysiology" by Ax (1964). The table of contents of this first issue of *Psychophysiology* reveals that in five of the eight original research articles the galvanic skin response (or electrodermal activity, as we would say today—see chapter 13) was the measure of interest, and there were no articles dealing with brain activity. By contrast, in a recent issue of *Psychophysiology* (November 1999), out of a total of thirteen articles, nine dealt with brain activity, and there were no articles in which electrodermal activity was measured. This change in the psychophysiological measures of interest to most (but not all) researchers is a reflection of a great increase in interest in cognitive functioning, plus improvements in the equipment used to record brain activity and the availability of computers and appropriate software to analyze the signals (see chapter 7).

In the remainder of this chapter, we will examine the past of psychophysiology, including the understanding of the electrical properties of the skin, and conclude with a brief discussion of the development of instrumentation.

### The Past of Psychophysiology

The early Greeks were interested in the location within the body of intellectual, emotional, and instinctual functioning. The philosopher Plato suggested that humans possessed a tripartite organization. He believed that rational faculties were located in the head. Passions were said to be located in the spinal marrow, which related them to the heart. The instincts—or lower appetites, as they were sometimes called—were said to be located in the spinal cord below the diaphragm, where they could influence the liver. There were parallels to Plato's system outside the Mediterranean area. In other parts of the world, the body was also thought of as being organized into different functional entities (e.g., chakras in the metaphysics of India) that performed differential psychological and physiological functions with respect to the development of the individual and the utilization of energy. In all of this philosophical investigation, there was little of what we today refer to as experimentation. Because of his belief that our senses deceive us, Plato rejected the idea of experimentation and placed pure thought above empirical observation as the means to achieve knowledge. In a vein similar to Plato's, Chinese science and medicine rejected dissection as a method that would lead to meaningful answers, relying instead on more holistic concepts of human physiology and functioning.

Yet there is evidence of a sort of psychophysiology before the Renaissance. Mesulam and Perry (1972) have shown, through a reexamination of texts from the third century B.C. to the eleventh century A.D., that there was considerable empirical sophistication in the writings of Erasistratos, Galen, and Ibn Sina.

Erasistratos, a physician during the time of Alexander, is credited with the following example of clinical psychophysiological observation. A general of the time married. The general's son by a previous marriage fell in love with the same woman (his stepmother) but, realizing that his love could not be brought out into the open, he resolved not to show his feelings. The boy then became ill and almost died. After a number of other doctors had failed to help the boy, Erasistratos worked with him and decided that the physical problems must be related to a problem of the mind. This conclusion, though accurate, was not surprising because contemporary medicine held that the mind and body affected each other. What is interesting from our standpoint is the method Erasistratos used to determine the source of the boy's problem. The technique illustrates an early study in lie detection. Erasistratos observed the reactions of the boy as various people came to his room. In a later account of this episode, Plutarch reported that certain signs—"stammering speech, sudden sweats, irregular palpitations of the heart"—were all present in the boy whenever the stepmother came to see him. Thus, Erasistratos realized and correctly diagnosed the problem as being due to the relationship between the boy and his stepmother. Mesulam and Perry remind us that Erasistratos was actually an early psychophysiologist developing a theory of stimulus-response specificity, a concept which will be discussed in chapter 5.

Galen, a second-century physician who is often thought of as a father of modern physiology, reported a similar case of lovesickness he diagnosed based on the subject's irregular pulse when she heard the name of her lover. A tenth-century example of these same psychophysiological principles is found in the work of Ibn Sina (Avicenna), who is sometimes referred to as the Persian Galen. Again, Ibn Sina utilized the method of elevated pulse rate to determine the person with whom one was in love.

### Understanding the Electrical Properties of the Skin

It was not until the end of the eighteenth century and the experiments of Luigi Galvani in Italy that the stage was set for the further development of psychophysiology (Hoff, 1936). Galvani's contribution was the demonstration that animals produce electricity that originates within the organism itself. Before this time, it was known that muscles of a frog, for example, would contract when connected to an electrical source, but it was not known that the muscles were capable of producing an electrical impulse of their own.

Galvani's research, together with the demonstration of the effect of applying electricity to paralyzed muscles, led to much speculation concerning how electricity could improve people's health. One theory suggested that diseases could be diagnosed by measuring changes in the distribution of electrical current in the body. (It is interesting to note that a similar theory is presently offered as the basis of acupuncture.) A second theory stated that there was a connection between electricity, animal magnetism, suggestibility, and hysteria. In particular, it was thought that through the utilization of a magnet, a hysterical symptom such as functional paralysis of an arm could be transferred to the opposite side of the body and the originally affected side thus restored to normal functioning. This was referred to as "transfert" by Charcot. It was through experimentation with this phenomenon that Vigouroux first observed skin resistance level changes. (For an up-to-date discussion of skin resistance and other aspects of electrodermal activity, see chapter 13.) Vigouroux measured skin resistance while the hysterical symptom was transferred from side to side. The hysterical symptom observed was a loss of sensitivity in part of the body, classically referred to as a conversion reaction or hysterical anesthesia. When the anesthesia was transferred from one side of the body to the other, Vigouroux noted that skin resistance levels taken from the insensitive side of the body were higher than those of the normally functioning side. After a number of these alternations, the skin resistance of each side of the body remained similar. Thus Vigouroux may have provided us with the first documentation of the habituation of skin resistance, that is, the diminution of a response to repeated stimulation (see chapter 5).

Féré, another early worker in this field, was also interested in Charcot's theory of hysteria. Before turning to the electrical properties of the skin, Féré performed research that utilized a hand dynamometer. In these studies he noted the pressure on the dynamometer as hysterics were presented with either sensory stimulation or material of an emotionally arousing nature. His apparent goal in these studies was to obtain some measure of the excitation of the nervous system. To this end, he later undertook another set of studies in which a current was applied to the anterior surface of the forearm of subjects as they were presented with emotional and sensory stimulation. In these studies, Féré measured the change in current flow as a function of the stimuli. Thus Féré reported in 1888 the first study of skin resistance responses. In addition, work was also being performed on skin conductance by Hermann, Tarchanoff, Sticker, Sommer, and others. The interested reader may consult Neumann and Blanton (1970) for a brief history and an excellent bibliography. At this time, we will turn to the experiments of Mueller, Veraguth, and Jung, which helped bring international attention to the study of skin resistance. As is often the case in science, similar or identical discoveries are made throughout the world by scientists working independently of one another. This was the case with Mueller, a Swiss engineer, who observed that changes in skin resistance appeared to correlate with changes in psychological state. Mueller consulted with Veraguth, a neurologist, and each independently wrote a series of papers on the subject, apparently without any knowledge of the earlier work in the area. Veraguth believed that he had found a new reflex, sensitive to emotional factors, that would be important in dealing with psychiatric problems.

It was in this connection that Veraguth influenced Jung, who combined the measure of skin resistance with a word-association procedure. Jung developed a procedure in which 100 words were said to an individual with the instruction, "Answer as quickly as possible with the first word that occurs to you." Jung timed the responses and then repeated the list (Jung, 1910). From this procedure, Jung sought to identify areas of the person's life which were emotionally important. In one series of experiments (Jung, 1907; Peterson and Jung, 1907; Ricksher and Jung, 1908), Jung and his colleagues studied the skin resistance responses of normal and abnormal populations. He also examined changes in respiration that were concomitant with the skin resistance response. In the last study just cited, Jung concluded that skin resistance responses were related to attention to the stimulus and the ability to associate it with previous occurrences, either conscious or unconscious. He also stated that physical stimuli elicit a greater response than psychological ones and that the reaction is greater in normal populations than in pathological ones.

### Instrumentation

The first instrument capable of reproducing a continuous record of a rapidly changing bioelectrical event was the capillary electrometer developed in the 1870s by Marey (Geddes and Baker, 1968). This instrument consisted of a tube filled with sulfuric acid and mercury. The electrical activity would change the shape of the mercury meniscus, and through the use of high-intensity light the variations in the contour of the meniscus would form the basis for recording. This was the first instrument to record and display the electrical activity of a frog's heart in the 1880s; the recording was made by Sir John Burdon-Sanderson. In 1887, Waller first recorded the electrical activity from the human heart using electrodes on the skin.

Although the capillary electrometer stimulated research in the recording of bioelectrical events, there were problems with the device. These problems prompted Einthoven—who is known as the father of electrocardiography—to develop a better device for recording electrical activity, the *string galvanometer*. This instrument proved to be reliable, and even though it was developed in the 1900s it was not fully replaced until the 1940s. A string galvanometer can be seen in the National Museum of American History at the Smithsonian Institution in Washington, D.C., along with some later devices for measuring the electrical activity of the heart.

In the 1920s additional physiological responses from human beings were recorded, and research and clinical interest soon followed. In 1929 Berger reported the first human electroencephalogram (EEG), which measured electrical activity from the brain. Berger not only named the EEG, he was also the first to report the alpha rhythm and beta rhythm. (See chapter 7 for more about brain wave activity.) In his early recording, he pushed platinum wires into the scalp. Later he placed plate electrodes on the front and back of the head and utilized the Einthoven string galvanometer. For a time, he also tried placing a silver spoon in the subject's mouth as the reference electrode, but later he abandoned the idea. In his work, Berger demonstrated EEG changes related to eye opening, large-scale stimuli, and mental activity and attention. He also observed the EEG in brain-damaged individuals. Within ten to fifteen years, the EEG had become a clinical tool utilizing multichannel ink writing instruments. With the introduction of the vacuum tube and then the transistor, psychophysiological recording was soon to become readily available as both a clinical and research tool.

The field of psychophysiological instrumentation has grown at a tremendous rate, especially since the introduction of the integrated circuit and the personal computer (PC). In many laboratories, the ink-writing polygraph has been replaced by a PC equipped with an analog to digital (A/D) board and data acquisition and analysis software. (See chapter 3 for more about instrumentation.)

This revolution in instrumentation has brought with it a change in the skills needed by the psychophysiologist. At one time, every psychophysiologist had to construct electronic circuits for particular recording needs, and even the electrodes had to be constructed by hand for each application. Today commercially available equipment is excellent and extremely reliable. With less emphasis on required electronic skills, the psychophysiologist has more time to devote to theoretical and empirical work related to the interaction of psychological and physiological factors.

References to the specific material covered in the following chapters are provided at the end of each chapter, but some more general sources of information about psychophysiology are also available. Andreassi (1995), in the third edition of his text, "Psychophysiology: Human Behavior and the Physiological Response," provides many excellent examples of applications of the psychophysiological recording techniques covered in this book. Hugdahl (1995) reviews numerous studies in the area of cognitive psychophysiology in his book, *Psychophysiology: The Mind-Body Perspective.* A more advanced treatment of the concepts and techniques used in psychophysiological recording can be found in Cacioppo and Tassinary (1990), *Principles of Psychophysiology: Physical, Social, and Inferential Elements.* A new *Handbook of Psychophysiology* (Cacioppo, Tassinary, & Berntson, 2000) is available. The URL of the web-page for the Society for Psychophysiological Research is http://www.sprweb.org; the site has a variety of information about psychophysiology and about the society, including information about the annual meeting and the society's journal, *Psychophysiology.* Other journals devoted to psychophysiological research include the *International Journal of Psychophysiology* and the *Journal of Psychophysiology.*

*References*

Andreassi, J. L. (1995). *Psychophysiology: Human behavior and physiological response* (3rd ed.). Hillsdale, NJ: Erlbaum.

Ax, A. F. (1964). Goals and methods of psychophysiology. *Psychophysiology, 1,* 8–25.

Cacioppo, J. T., & Tassinary, L. G. (1990). *Principles of psychophysiology: Physical, social, and inferential elements.* Cambridge: Cambridge University Press.

Cacioppo, J. T., Tassinary, L. G., & Berntson, G. G. (2000). *Handbook of psychophysiology.* Cambridge: Cambridge University Press.

Darrow, C. W. (1964). Psychophysiology, yesterday, today, and tomorrow. *Psychophysiology, 1,* 4–7.

Fahrenberg, J., & Myrtek, M. (Eds.) (1996). *Ambulatory assessment. Computer-assisted psychological and psychophysiological methods in monitoring and field studies.* Seattle: Hogrefe & Huber.

Hugdahl, K. (1995). *Psychophysiology: The mind-body perspective.* Cambridge, MA: Harvard University Press.

Geddes, L. A., & Baker, L. E. (1968). *Principles of applied biomedical instrumentation.* New York: Wiley.

Hoff, H. (1936). Galvani and the pregalvanian electrophysiologists. *Annals of Science, 1,* 147–172.

Jung, C. G. (1907). On the psychological relations of the association experiment. *Journal of Abnormal Psychology, 7,* 247–255.

Jung, C. G. (1910). The association method. *American Journal of Psychology, 21,* 219–269.

Mesulam, M., & Perry, J. (1972). The diagnosis of love-sickness: Experimental psychophysiology without the polygraph. *Psychophysiology, 9,* 546–551.

Neumann, E., & Blanton, R. (1970). The early history of electrodermal research. *Psychophysiology, 6,* 453–475.

Peterson, F., & Jung, C. G. (1907). Psychophysical investigations with the galvanometer and insane individuals. *Brain, 30,* 143–182.

Ricksher, C., & Jung, C. G. (1908). Further investigations on the galvanic phenomenon and respiration in normal and insane individuals. *Journal of Abnormal Psychology, 2,* 189–217.

Stern, J. A. (1964). Towards a definition of psychophysiology. *Psychophysiology, 1,* 90–91.

# 2

# Neurons and Muscles

*The Sources of Psychophysiological Recordings*

The bodily responses that are the subject of psychophysiological study originate as electrochemical changes in *neurons* (nerve cells), muscles, and gland cells. These signals spread from their sources through the body to the skin surface, appearing to a recording electrode on the body surface in a somewhat altered form. Understanding the genesis of bioelectric potentials will help in interpreting the surface potentials and serve as a reminder that whatever their relation to behavior, psychophysiological responses reflect the functioning of neurons, muscles, and glands.

The nervous system controls the bodily functions measured by psychophysiologists, including muscle action, organ function, and glandular activity. For example, the coordinated contraction of thousands of skeletal muscle cells moves us through our environment; enables us to react to its changes; and is the mechanism of singing, smiling, sitting, and eating. Cardiac muscle cells pump blood to the lungs and through the body; smooth muscle cells move food through the digestive system from one end to the other and generate the uterine forces which move the fetus from gestation to birth. All these activities require coordinated action of muscle cells. They must be coordinated with each other, both within and between muscles, as well as with other organ systems and environmental events. The random twitchings of thousands of cells could produce neither effective action nor sustained life. A rapid communication system is provided by the nervous system, a group of cells specialized for the transmission of information (see figure 2.1). Neurons with their branching processes pervade the body, interconnecting sense organs with muscle and gland systems. Events occurring at one place in the body are quickly and reliably reported to structures elsewhere. This conveying of information throughout the body is elaborate in complex organisms, where billions of nerve cells ensure that the simplest muscular reflex is coor-

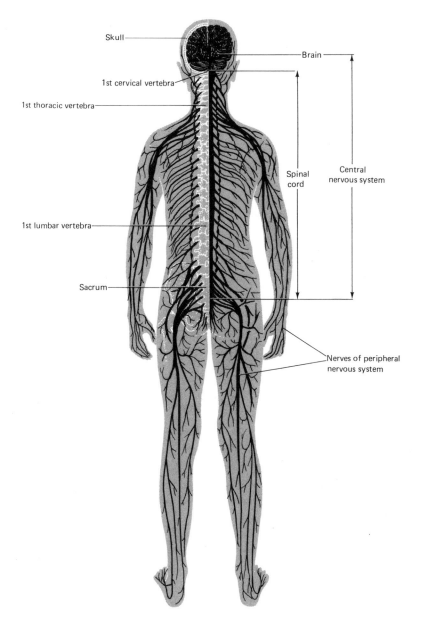

Figure 2.1. The nervous system. Redrawn with permission from A. W. Ham, 1974, *Histology* (7th ed.). Philadelphia: Lippincott.

dinated with posture, other reflexes, organ states, events in the environment, and the experience of the organism.

## Organization of the Nervous System

There are at least 100 billion nerve cells in the human nervous system (Guyton, 1987); some knowledge of their organization is useful in understanding their function. Neurons are usually found in bundles that reflect their origin and their destination. These bundles, called nerves in the *peripheral nervous system* (PNS) and tracts within the *central nervous system* (CNS), may include only a few neurons or millions of them. The PNS includes all neurons outside the bony enclosures of the spinal column and skull, and the CNS is composed of all those cells inside it. Note that this is a distinction of convenience because the PNS and CNS are not really separate systems. Indeed, some neurons are contained partly in the CNS and partly in the PNS.

Neurons are somewhat oddly shaped cells of the body. A schematized neuron, is depicted in figure 2.2. The receiving end of a neuron is equipped with *dendrites* that accept chemical messages from other neurons or, in the case of sensory neurons that generate a signal within the neuron, when a sensory stimulus is received (e.g., a dendrite transmits information about touch when pressure deforms it). Dendrites extend from the neuron's *cell body*, which contains the genetic material and the energy-generating machinery of the cell. Extending away from the cell body is a long process called the *axon*; the axon ends in *axon terminals*. Signals internal to a neuron typically pass from the dendrites to the cell body to the axon and finally to the axon terminals. At the axon terminals, chemical substances called *neurotransmitters* are released into the extracellular fluid. Neurotransmitters diffuse across the extracellular space be-

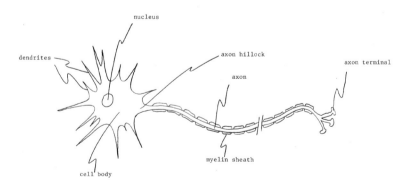

Figure 2.2. Major components of a neuron. The double slash marks through the axon indicate that the full length of the axon has not been drawn.

tween two neurons and are received at receptors on the dendrites of a nearby neuron. If the neurotransmitter finds a matching receptor, then an electrical change is initiated in the neuron receiving the chemical message. We will discuss the function of these neuronal components in more detail later.

Neurons can be functionally distinguished by the direction in which they conduct impulses. Neurons conducting impulses toward a particular structure are *afferent* neurons (often the point of reference is the CNS); those conducting impulses away from a particular structure are *efferent* neurons. Functionally independent afferent and efferent neurons, such as those conducting sensory information to the CNS, and motor information away from the CNS can be, and often are, found in the same nerve bundle.

### Sensory Systems

Sensory neurons, which translate sensory signals such as light or pressure into neural signals send information from sensory receptors to the CNS. Sensory neurons usually do not synapse before entering the CNS; this means that a single neuron transmits information from a sensory receptor in a muscle, the skin, or an internal organ directly to the spinal cord or brain; a notable exception occurs in the retina of the eye. Once information reaches the spinal cord or the brain, other neurons convey that information to sites both within the CNS and, in some cases, to motor neurons leading back out of the CNS. The nervous system does not connect muscles directly to other muscles or glands, nor does it conduct sensory information from the environment directly to the muscles. Rather, the sensory information goes first to the CNS, from which it is redistributed both inside and outside the CNS. This arrangement provides the capacity for integrating incoming sensory signals with conditions elsewhere in the body where the CNS acts as the "executive system" in charge of coordinating action and function throughout the body.

### Motor Systems

Anatomically the motor neurons can be divided into two subsystems, the somatic motor system and the autonomic nervous system. Although historically the autonomic subdivision of the PNS was considered a motor system, a considerable number of sensory fibers are present within autonomic nerve bundles (Loewy, 1990). Thus, the autonomic nervous system is more correctly considered both a motor and sensory system for control of, and feedback from, the internal organs and glands. However, because much more is known about the efferent function of the ANS, we will only consider here its role as an efferent system for control of organs and glands.

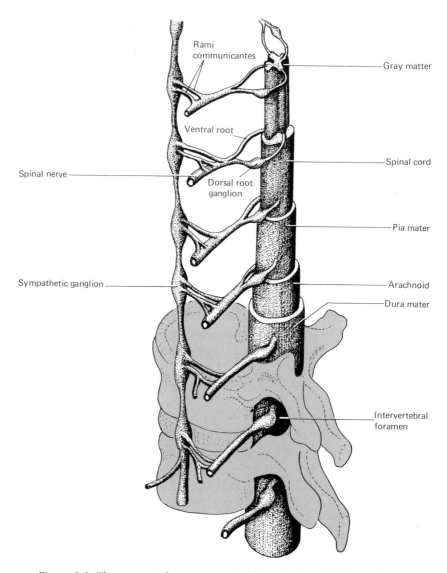

Figure 2.3. The segmental arrangement of the spinal cord. Redrawn by permission from E. Gardner, (1975), *Fundamentals of neurology* (6th ed.), Philadelphia: Saunders.

*Somatic System.* The *somatic nervous system* is composed of efferent neurons that project out of the CNS and innervate the skeletal musculature. The dendrites of motor neurons that receive incoming messages are found within the central horn (i.e., gray matter) of the spinal cord at each spinal segment (there is one segment for each vertebra; see figure 2.3). The motor neurons in each spinal nerve extend without synapse to a group of striate (skeletal) muscles at approximately the level of the vertebral segment from which the neuronal processes emerged. The axons of each motor neuron run close to one another in the spinal nerve and then separate from one another near the target muscle, so that a single motor neuron typically terminates at the motor end plates of several muscle cells. Each motor neuron and the group of muscle cells innervated by that motor neuron is called a *motor unit*—all the muscle cells will necessarily contract together in response to action potentials originating in the motor neuron. In the somatic motor system, this route from the CNS to the motor unit is called the final common path, reflecting the invariant nature of the system once an action potential has been generated in the spinal motor neuron.

Considering this arrangement of motor units, one might predict that where there is fine control of muscular action, the motor units would be small when compared to those muscles over which we have relatively crude control. Sure enough, motor units are much smaller in the muscles controlling eye movements than in the large muscles of the back. This difference in control is referred to as the *size principle*. Not only do smaller motor units control fewer muscle fibers and thus confer finer muscle control than do large motor units, but smaller motor units also are recruited faster than larger motor units. This faster recruitment of smaller motor units allows for movements to be initiated gradually and smoothly, which is particularly important when large muscle masses are activated (Guyton & Hall, 1996).

*Autonomic System.* The *autonomic nervous system* (ANS) consists of two major branches or divisions, the *sympathetic nervous system* and the *parasympathetic nervous system*. The two divisions of the ANS are anatomically quite different than the somatic system. Efferent neuronal fibers from the somatic system exit the CNS and innervate a muscle without synapse. Efferent fibers from the ANS, on the other hand, emerge from the CNS and synapse once outside the CNS before reaching the target organ or gland. The anatomical structure formed by the synapses between the neurons exiting the spinal cord and the dendrites and cell bodies of receiving neurons is called a *ganglion* (plural is *ganglia*). Ganglia for the sympathetic nervous system lie in a chain near the spinal cord and vertebral column. Ganglia for the parasympathetic nervous system typically lie in the wall of the target organ. Thus, even the anatomy of the two major autonomic branches is quite dissimilar. We also now recognize a third division of the ANS: the enteric nervous system, which regulates much of the function of the gastrointestinal system.

*Sympathetic division.* The sympathetic division is composed of those neurons that originate within the thoracic and lumbar segments of the spinal cord and project to ganglia lying along the vertebral column just outside the cord (see figure 2.4). Because of its anatomical arrangement,

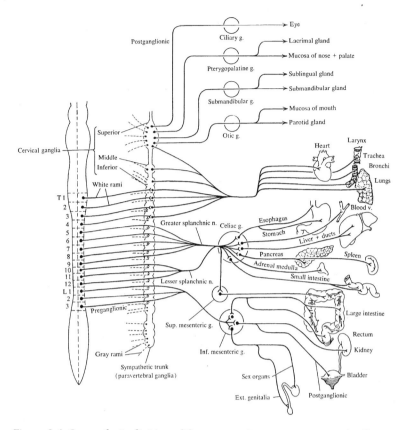

Figure 2.4. Sympathetic division of the autonomic nervous system. This figure illustrates the preganglionic axons exiting the spinal cord, the ganglia making up the sympathetic chain, and the postganglionic fibers innervating target organs and glands. Figure used with permission from B. Pansky, D. J. Allen, & G. C. Budd, 1988, *Review of neuroscience* (2nd ed.), New York: Macmillan.

the sympathetic division has also been called the thoracolumbar system. There is a ganglion through which efferent fibers of the sympathetic system pass for each spinal segment from the first thoracic to the third lumbar segment. Many of these ganglia are interconnected to form the chain of ganglia on each side of the vertebral column. Efferent neurons from the spinal cord (i.e., preganglionic neurons) that enter the sympathetic chain may synapse at the same segmental level where they exit from the cord, or they may extend up or down the chain to enter other ganglia, or they may even pass directly through the chain without synapse. The efferent fibers leaving the sympathetic chain (also known as postganglionic neurons) innervate smooth muscles and glands in the skin, eyes, mucous membranes, and viscera. Most postganglionic sympathetic fibers extend directly from cell bodies in the chain ganglia to a target organ. However, postganglionic fibers innervating the smooth muscles and glands of the abdomen and pelvic area originate in ganglia lying near the sympathetic chain (e.g., the celiac and inferior mesenteric ganglia; see figure 2.4). The rule is that there is a preganglionic and a postganglionic fiber providing autonomic input to a target organ; one interesting exception is the case of the adrenal medulla. A single preganglionic neuron extends without synapse directly to the adrenal medulla, where norepinephrine and epinephrine are released into the blood stream as hormones (Edwards, 1990). This is a somewhat unusual mode of delivery for the ANS, where substances are typically released as neurotransmitters onto a postsynaptic cell. However, the secretory cells that release norepinephrine and epinephrine are developmentally derived from nervous system cells, and function essentially as a specialized type of postganglionic neuron (Guyton & Hall, 1996).

The neurotransmitter released at the ganglia onto the dendrites of the postganglionic neuron is *acetylcholine*. Here, acetylcholine activates cholinergic receptors of the nicotinic subtype (which, as the name implies, respond to nicotine). The neurotransmitter released by the terminals of the sympathetic postganglionic neurons onto target organs and glands is norepinephrine, with the exception of the eccrine sweat glands, where acetylcholine is the transmitter (see chapter 13 for a description). Thus, the norepinephrine released into the bloodstream as a hormone by the adrenal medulla activates most targets innervated by the sympathetic division.

*Parasympathetic division.* The second major division of the ANS is the craniosacral, or parasympathetic division. The parasympathetic division is composed of preganglionic neurons whose cell bodies lie in the brain stem and in the sacral segments of the spinal cord, and synapse onto postganglionic neurons in or near the target organ (see figure 2.5). Postganglionic neurons in the cranial division innervate the eyes, the mucosa of the nose and mouth, the salivary glands, the heart, the lungs and bronchi, and the abdominal organs. Postganglionic neurons in the sacral division innervate the genitalia and organs of the pelvic cavity, such as the bladder and bowel. As with the sympathetic system, the neurotransmitter released by the preganglionic fibers onto the postganglionic dendrites is acetylcholine, which activates cholinergic receptors of the nicotinic subtype. As in the somatic system, the neurotransmitter at the terminals of the postganglionic neurons in the parasympathetic division is acetylcholine, and here it activates cholinergic receptors of the muscarinic subtype.

The parasympathetic division innervates many of the same target organs and glands as the sympathetic system, although the overlap is not complete. When both divisions of the autonomic nervous system innervate the same target, we say that the target is dually innervated. This is a common pattern in autonomic anatomy. Often, activation of the two

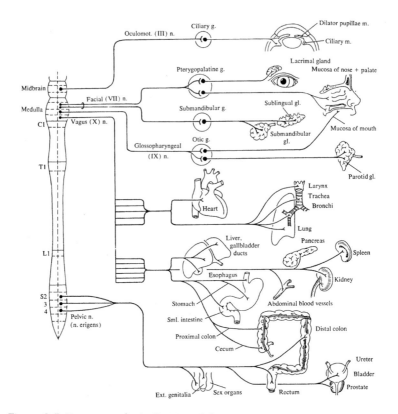

Figure 2.5. Parasympathetic division of the autonomic nervous system. This figure illustrates the preganglionic axons exiting the brain and spinal cord and entering ganglia. Postganglionic axons leaving ganglia and entering a target organ or gland are also shown. Where ganglia are located very near or within the target organ, the postganglionic cell bodies and axons are not shown. Figure used with permission from B. Pansky, D. J. Allen & G. C. Budd, 1988, *Review of neuroscience* (2nd ed.), New York: Macmillan.

branches exerts differential effects on the target organ. For example, the heart receives input from both the sympathetic and parasympathetic branches of the ANS. Increasing sympathetic activation of the heart leads to an increased rate of beating of the heart. Conversely, reducing activity in the sympathetic branch innervating the heart causes the heart beat to slow. At the heart, the parasympathetic system acts in a manner opposite to the sympathetic. Thus, increasing parasympathetic activation of the heart decreases the heart rate and decreasing parasympathetic activation increases the heart rate. It should be kept in mind that both branches of the ANS can be tonically active (meaning that there is some ongoing activity in the nerves) even when the body is at rest. This permits both increases and decreases in activity in *either* branch to make changes in the functional state of a given target organ. It used to be assumed that when activity in one branch increased, that activity in the other autonomic branch necessarily decreased (referred to as a reciprocal mode of ANS control). This is not always true, however. Sometimes activity in one autonomic branch increases or decreases, with no change in the activity of the other branch (uncoupled mode of ANS control), or activity in both branches can simultaneously increase or decrease (coactivational mode of ANS control). These three modes of ANS control—reciprocal, uncoupled, and coactivational—can occur for any target organ receiving innervation from both autonomic branches. These multiple modes permit subtle changes in the function of the target organ that are not possible with only reciprocal activation (see chapter 12 and Berntson, Cacioppo, & Quigley, 1991, for more discussion of this issue). Table 2.1 depicts the usual effects of the *activation* of the sympathetic and parasympathetic divisions on various organs.

## Function of Nerve and Muscle Cells

Nerve cells and muscle cells are alike in two important ways; they are elongated and they are excitable. Elongation refers to the long, narrow shape of nerve and muscle cells. Cells are called excitable when a stimulus that occurs at one point on the cell causes an electrical disturbance that spreads over much or all of the cell. These two properties combine to create the distribution of local events over large areas and great distances. Indeed, neural excitation may be propagated for a meter or more in some nerve cells.

### Excitability: Resting Potential and Action Potential

When nerve and muscle cells are inactive, an electrical potential can be observed across the cell membrane. The inside of the cell is approximately $-90$ mV compared to the outside (see figure 2.6). This means that unlike charges have been separated, with positive charges lying along the outside of the cell membrane and negative charges along the inside of the cell membrane. The fact that charges are separated also means that there is a capacity to perform work. The resting nerve or muscle cell is like a tiny flashlight battery in which charges are held apart, to be used when a path between the positive and negative charges is created. The separation of charges is termed *polarization*, and the resulting steady electrical potential between the inside and outside of excitable cells is called the *resting potential*.

The resting potential is due to the resting cell's permeability to potassium $(K^+)$, the cell's relative impermeability to ions such as sodium

Table 2.1. Effects of the Autonomic Nervous System on Selected Target Organs and Glands

| Structure | Function | Increased Parasympathetic Activity | Increased Sympathetic Activity |
|---|---|---|---|
| Eyes: Iris | Control of light to the eye | | |
| -radial muscle | | —[a] | Contraction (pupil dilates) |
| -sphincter muscle | | Contraction (pupil constricts) | —[a] |
| Eyes: Ciliary muscle (attached to the lens) | Accommodation | Constriction (near vision) | Relaxation (far vision) |
| Nasal glands | Secretion | Increased secretion | —[a] |
| Lacrimal glands | Tear production | Increased secretion | —[a] |
| Salivary glands | Saliva production | Increased potassium and water secretion (profuse, thin secretion) | Some increase in potassium, water and amylase secretion (viscous secretion) |
| Gastrointestinal | Muscle tone and motility | Increased motility and tone | Some decrease in motility and tone |
| Pancreas (islets) | Insulin secretion | Increased release | Decreased ($\alpha_2$-adrenergic) and increased ($\beta_2$-adrenergic) release |
| Heart: S-A node | Rate control | Slows rate | Increases rate |
| Heart: atria and ventricles | Contractility control | Some decrease in contractility | Increase in contractility |
| Bronchi of lungs | Bronchial muscle tone | Contraction and narrowing of bronchi | Relaxation and dilation of bronchi |

| Organ | Parameter | Parasympathetic | Sympathetic |
|---|---|---|---|
| Adrenal medulla | Secretion of catecholamines (epinephrine & norepinephrine) | —[a] | Secretion of catecholamines |
| Arterioles: skeletal muscle | Arterial tone | Slight dilation | Both constriction and dilation |
| Arterioles: skin | Arterial tone | —[a] | Constriction |
| Sweat glands | Sweat production | —[a] | Increased sweating |
| Pilomotor muscles | Erection of hair | —[a] | Initiation of "goose flesh" or "goose bumps" |
| Bladder: muscle wall | Muscle tone | Contraction | Relaxation |
| Bladder: sphincter | Muscle tone | Relaxation | Contraction |
| Male genitalia | Sexual behavior | Erection | Emission & ejaculation |

*Note:* The table is organized with organs and glands innervated by the cranial portion of the parasympathetic division at the top, the effectors innervated by the thoracolumbar (sympathetic) division in the middle, and the effectors innervated by the sacral portion of the parasympathetic division at the bottom of the table. Thus, the table roughly reflects the anatomical organization of the ANS. The horizontal spaces in the table separate the cranial, thoracolumbar and sacral divisions. Information in the table was compiled from Berne & Levy (1998), Guyton & Hall (1996), and Loewy & Spyer (1990).

[a] Indicates that there is no known functional effect of the branch indicated.

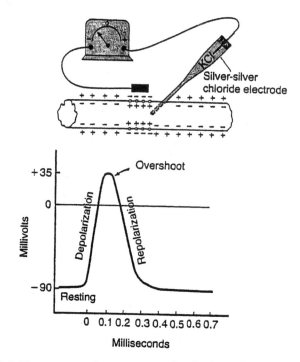

Figure 2.6. The resting and action potentials. The figure illustrates the resting potential of a neuron (approx. −90 mV), and the rapid depolarization and repolarization that occurs when an action potential is fired. Above the illustration of the potentials is a depiction of the way in which these potentials are measured, using an electrode that impales the axon and records the electrical potential of the inside of the cell relative to the outside of the cell. Figure used with permission from A. C. Guyton & J. E. Hall, 1996, *Textbook of medical physiology* (9th ed.), Philadelphia: Saunders.

($Na^+$), and an energy-requiring $Na^+-K^+$ pump in the cell's membrane which helps to maintain the relative negativity of the inner surface of the cell membrane. The cell membrane is semipermeable, meaning that some substances can pass through the membrane whereas others cannot. The major contributor to the resting potential is the *$Na^+-K^+$ pump* which requires metabolic energy and pumps 3 $Na^+$ ions out of the cell while simultaneously bringing 2 $K^+$ ions into the cell. As the pump works, there is a greater accumulation of positive ions on the outside of the cell and a relative negativity on the inside of the cell (i.e., fewer positive ions). Together, these factors result in a cell with the potential to do the work of the nervous system or create muscular activity. For a more comprehensive description of the basis of the resting potential, see Guyton and Hall (1996) or Berne and Levy (1998).

When the resting potential of the cell is reduced slightly at a point on the membrane (i.e., the inside of the cell becomes more positive relative to the outside), several local events occur. First, the membrane momentarily becomes more permeable to sodium, so that sodium ions begin to enter the cell from outside. Local currents are then created as ions move across the membrane. However, if the current flow is small (only a few millivolts), the disturbance will remain localized and likely will not spread to excite the entire cell. However, if a stronger stimulus (i.e., a larger decrease in membrane potential or depolarization) is applied to the membrane, this creates a very different effect. If the depolarization reaches a certain level, termed *threshold* (in the neighborhood of a 20–40 mV reduction in transmembrane potential), then the membrane becomes very permeable to sodium, which enters the cell quickly. This results in a rapid change across the membrane such that the inside of the neuron briefly becomes positively charged. The increase in sodium permeability, large sodium influx, and quick reduction of negative potential in the cell occurs explosively and ends only when all of the energy stored at that point on the membrane has been exhausted. When the cell membrane becomes briefly positive, then the approximately 90 mV resting potential has been discharged.

Just after the influx of sodium, sodium inactivation gates close and the membrane again becomes highly impermeable to sodium. Subsequently, the $Na^+-K^+$ pump begins to force sodium out of the cell in exchange for potassium ions that enter the cell. This mechanism restores the resting potential. The explosive chain of events during which the potential across the membrane is discharged is called the *action potential* of excitable cells and is the mechanism of excitation in nerve and muscle cells. The relatively large local currents produced by initiation of an action potential are sufficient to propagate this potential to nearby portions of the cell by reducing the membrane potential there to threshold value, and thereby triggering an action potential. This is analogous to the burning of a fuse on a firecracker, where the burning fuse successively ignites all along the length of the fuse. Interestingly, the action potential is undiminished as it moves over the cell, because energy is stored all along the length of the cell. As a result, the excitation of a given nerve cell is uniform each time an action potential is fired; this excitation is independent of the size or physical nature of the stimulus, as long as depolarization exceeds the threshold. The fact that the action potential is either (a) initiated when depolarization reaches threshold or (b) not initiated when changes in polarity are below threshold is referred to as the *all-or-none principle*. This principle implies that if the stimulus is great enough to cause an action potential, the cell will be completely depolarized, regardless of further increases in the amplitude of the stimulus. On the other hand, a subthreshold stimulus will produce only local changes that are not propagated along the length of the cell.

The consequences of action potentials are quite different in muscle and nerve cells. We will first examine muscle cells and the activity of the three types of muscles found in the body—striate, smooth, and cardiac—and then return to our discussion of nerve cells.

## Muscles

*Groups of Muscle Cells: Muscles.*   Acting alone, single muscle cells would be incapable of producing the great tensions required to move the long bones and to support the skeleton against the force of gravity. In fact, muscle cells are ordinarily arranged in groups, with like cells having the same function. These groups, of course, are muscles. Muscles are of two very different kinds—*striate* (skeletal) and *smooth*—with cardiac (or heart) muscle exhibiting some of the properties of each. Cardiac muscle is striated like skeletal muscle but operates as a syncytium, or interconnected unit, like most smooth muscle does.

*Striate muscle.* Striate, or striped muscle is sometimes called *skeletal muscle* because it attaches to the bones and is responsible for support and movement of skeletal body parts. Striate muscle is relatively fast-acting, although there is a wide variation in contraction speed from the slow muscles of the back to the fast muscles of the eyelid. Not all striate muscles are attached to bones at both ends. For example, the muscles of facial expression arise from and attach to connective tissue; thus smiling and frowning do not involve the skeleton. However, most striate muscles are arranged around bones, arising from tendons and ligaments on one side of a joint and inserting into bone on the other side of the joint, so that muscle shortening produces tension across the joint. If tension is sufficient, there will be movement of bone around the joint. Due to their anatomical placement, other muscles may oppose this action, so their action can prevent movement or move the bone in the opposite direction. At complex joints such as the ankle, hip, wrist, and neck, many muscles surround the joint, providing support and movement in many directions.

The cells of striate muscle are electrically insulated from each other. As a result, an action potential spreading over a cell does not affect neighboring cells. This means that both the initiation of contraction and coordinated contractions of groups of muscle cells must come from outside the muscle by way of the nervous system. Striate muscle deprived of its nerve supply is completely relaxed unless action potentials are artificially generated by electrical or chemical stimulation. Paralysis following severe damage to the spinal cord is an example of intact, otherwise healthy muscles that are incapable of generating tension because they are receiving no external input.

The cellular basis of striate or skeletal muscle contraction is relatively well understood and so we will explore it in some detail. The skeletal muscle cell, or fiber, is composed of slender myofibrils. Each fibril is made up of tiny filaments, which are the contracting units of the cell. These filaments, which lie longitudinally within the fiber, are of two kinds: actin and myosin. In a noncontracted state, adjacent actin and myosin filaments overlap slightly but are not bound to one another. When contraction is initiated, bonds between the two types of filaments are quickly made, the fibers are pulled alongside one another such that the filaments overlap to a greater extent, and then the bond is broken. This process is often described as a kind of "ratcheting" movement with repeated sequences of bond formation, pulling together of the fibers, and breaking of the bond as the muscle fibers become overlapped to a greater and greater extent with each sequence. As the two kinds of filaments slide alongside one another, the myofibril shortens along its longitudinal axis. When this occurs in many adjacent myofibrils it causes contraction or shortening of the entire muscle fiber.

Skeletal muscle contraction is initiated when a neuron sends a message to the muscle at the particular neuromuscular junction that is the point of contact between a nerve cell axon terminal and a muscle cell. Release of the neurotransmitter acetylcholine onto the muscle at the neuromuscular junction causes an action potential to be propagated in the muscle fibers. The muscle action potential then causes calcium to be released. The influx of calcium to the filaments begins a chemical reaction, part of which is used to initiate the ratcheting and sliding motion of the actin and myosin filaments. A thorough account of the contractile process may be found in Guyton and Hall (1996) or Berne and Levy (1998).

The time required for contraction varies greatly in different muscles, but it is always much longer than the action potential that precedes it. Even in relatively fast skeletal muscle, the contraction-relaxation sequence to a single stimulus may not be complete for 30–200 ms even though the action potential lasts only 1–5 ms. In addition, the action potential can be complete before contraction even begins.

Under normal circumstances the action potential is always of the same magnitude in a given cell, and it might be expected that the contractile response of the muscle cell would always be the same (i.e., that it would result in the same shortening or increase in tension). However, this is not always the case. If the relaxation phase following contraction is completed, then the tension produced by a succeeding action potential will indeed be similar. If, however, a second action potential is propagated before the previous contraction is complete, a further increase in tension results. The amount of increased tension depends on the interval between the two stimuli, with shorter intervals producing greater increases in tension. This effect, called *frequency summation*, continues as the frequency of stimulation increases, with each succeeding increase in frequency adding a diminishing amount of tension until further increases add no more tension (figure 2.7). At this point, the muscle cell is in a state of continuing maximal tension called *tetanus*. Thus, a single striate (skeletal) muscle cell is capable of finely graded contractions that depend

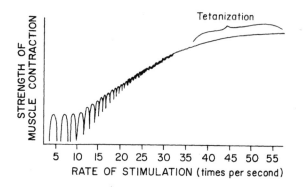

Figure 2.7. The process of tetanization. The figure demonstrates how tetanus develops in striate muscle as the frequency of stimulation of a muscle increases. Note that contraction is smooth and sustained once the rate of stimulation becomes sufficiently high. Figure used with permission from A. C. Guyton & J. E. Hall, 1996, *Textbook of medical physiology* (9th ed.), Philadelphia. Saunders.

on the rate at which action potentials are generated. Whereas striate muscle is capable of tetanic contraction, smooth muscle is not. Smooth muscle, such as that found in the stomach, can also sustain maximal tension, however, it uses a different mechanism than tetanization.

*Smooth muscle.* Smooth muscle is found in layers around the hollow organs of the gastrointestinal tract, around the uterus and bladder, and surrounding the arteries. Smooth muscle also controls constriction and dilation of the pupils and the limited action of some body hair (as when hair "stands on end" or you get "goose bumps"). Smooth muscle contracts slowly. An action potential may produce a complete contraction-relaxation cycle only after a second or two. There are two types of smooth muscle: multi-unit and unitary. Multi-unit smooth muscle operates much like striate muscle cells because each cell is physically separate from its neighboring cells and activation of single cells generally occurs when there is input from a neuron. In contrast, action potentials generated in unitary smooth muscle cells spread to other smooth muscle cells via *gap junctions* (low-resistence connections) that permit the spread of electrical current between cells. This ability to spread activation over a large number of cells means that a contraction in one part of a smooth muscle may, in effect, spread over the muscle with minimal or even no neural input. For example, hormones or mechanical changes (such as stretch) can produce smooth muscle contraction that is initiated without any neural input to the muscle.

In addition, the resting potential of some smooth muscle cells (particularly those of the gastrointestinal tract) fluctuates rhythmically. These spontaneous changes in the resting potential, called slow waves, can generate action potentials and hence contractions. Contraction of smooth muscle can be both initiated and maintained under local control as a result of spontaneous rhythmic variations and direct electrical conduction between cells.

*Cardiac muscle.* Cardiac muscle acts faster than smooth muscle, but the interconnection of cells is similar such that electrical activity can spread quickly over many cells. The heart has two regions of functionally interconnected muscle cells, the atrial syncytium and the ventricular syncytium. Syncytia are composed of cells connected by gap junctions. Thus, the muscle cells of the atrial syncytium conduct action potentials virtually simultaneously, as do the cells of the ventricular syncytium. There is, however, a slight delay between contraction of the atria and contraction of the ventricles because electrical current passes between these two syncytia via a specialized bundle of conducting fibers called the atrioventricular (A/V) bundle. This delay is important because it allows time for blood to move from the atria to the ventricles so that there is sufficient blood in the ventricles before contraction to move blood into the arterial system (see chapter 12 for more details).

### Neurons

*Conduction in a Neuron.* In individual nerve cells, an action potential is generated when a sufficient increase in positive potential occurs at the dendrites or cell body. At the point where the axon exits from the cell body is a portion of the axon known as the *axon hillock*, where changes in potential coming from all around the cell body and dendrites are summed and if threshold is reached, an action potential is generated. The rate at which the action potential is conducted down the axon depends on two factors: (a) the diameter of the axon, and (b) whether or not the axon is myelinated. Conduction speed is faster in large diameter axons than in small diameter ones, the speed being proportional to the square root of the diameter.

The other condition that greatly increases the speed of the impulse along the nerve fiber is the presence of a *myelin sheath*. Many nerve cells that conduct over long distances are individually encased in a sheath of fatty material called myelin. This sheath gives nerve tracts their characteristic white appearance. Indeed, areas of myelinated and unmyelinated fibers in the brain are termed white and gray matter, respectively. Myelin is highly resistive to the passage of current, so that the resting potential does not develop in myelinated areas. Indeed, if the entire axon were covered in myelin, no impulse would be able to be conducted because the sheath would prevent any current spread. However, the myelin sheath contains tiny gaps where the axon membrane is exposed (these gaps are only about 2–3 mm long). These gaps, called *nodes of Ranvier*, occur about every 1 mm along the axon and permit local current flows through one of these exposed sections of membrane, which then depolarizes the membrane to threshold at the next node thereby generating an action potential at the subsequent node. Thus, the impulse "jumps" across adjacent nodes of Ranvier along the length of the neuron. This action, termed *saltatory conduction*, greatly speeds conduction, since no time is spent depolarizing the membrane between the nodes. Indeed, the impulse moves about 40–80 times faster in a myelinated fiber than in an unmyelinated fiber of the same diameter. For example, Morell and Norton (1980) point out that a human spinal cord that contained only unmyelinated axons would need to be several *yards* in diameter to conduct impulses as quickly as it can in its normal, myelinated state. Conduction velocities as fast as 120 m/s (which is greater than the length of a football field in 1 s) can be observed in large diameter myelinated axons, whereas small, unmyelinated axons may propagate signals as slowly as 0.25 m/s (Guyton & Hall, 1996).

When the action potential reaches the end of the neuron, it causes a momentary release of neurotransmitters stored within the axon terminals. This process describes the action of single nerve cells; electrical events occurring at the receiving end of the cell cause the release of chemicals from the transmitting end of the cell. The interconnections of numerous neurons, with each other and with sense organs, muscles, and glands are the basis for the function of the nervous system.

*Communication between Neurons.* Until now, we have mostly described events along the length of the axons. But since we noted earlier that, once started, the action potential is unchanged as it passes down the axon, then it must be the processes happening at the synapses between the neurons that are responsible for the variety of our experience and the subtlety of our actions.

*Receptor or generator potentials.* In the sensory neurons, dendrites generate messages when receptors are activated by sensory stimuli. These messages can be in the form of stimuli that are mechanical (e.g., pressure or vibration), thermal (e.g., heat or cold), nociceptive (e.g., painful), electromagnetic (e.g., light), or chemical (e.g., taste or smell). These stimuli act on specialized receptors and generate a depolarizing potential or receptor potential across the receptor membrane. When a receptor potential is generated, there is a change in electrical potential of the neuron that is proportional to the amount of stimulation received (such a proportional response is called graded). An action potential may be initiated when graded receptor potentials from multiple sensory receptors are combined with other changes in potential coming in at points all over the cell. Therefore, sensory signals differ as a result of the degree of stimulation received at the sensory receptors and due to the number and frequency of action potentials generated, not because of differences between action potentials across various sensory systems. Thus, our knowledge of the world around us and within us is a function of our sensory receptors and their sensitivity.

*The synapse: EPSPs and IPSPs.* Most nerve cells terminate in the immediate vicinity of other nerve cells. The region where two neurons meet and where neurotransmission can take place between them is called a *synapse*. Adjacent neurons do not touch one another; instead there is a small space between them called a *synaptic cleft*. When an impulse arrives at the axon terminals, it does not "hop" the gap between the presynaptic and postsynaptic cells. Instead, an action potential in the presynaptic cell causes the release of a neurotransmitter from the axon terminals of that cell. The neurotransmitter then diffuses across the synaptic cleft and arrives at the membrane of the postsynaptic cell. The neurotransmitter next causes depolarization or hyperpolarization of the dendritic membrane of the postsynaptic cell. The effect of the neurotransmitter is determined by the chemical composition of the transmitter substance. Moreover, a neurotransmitter can be effective only if it finds a receptor whose structure matches the structure of the transmitter. If the neurotransmitter partially depolarizes the postsynaptic cell membrane, then an *excitatory postsynaptic potential* (EPSP) has occurred. It is excitatory because it moves the transmembrane voltage closer to threshold level, making the cell easier to excite. It is worth noting that the transmitter released by a single action potential from a single terminal is not sufficient to produce an action potential in a postsynaptic cell. The effect of multiple action potentials in many presynaptic cells is required to excite a postsynaptic cell. Some neurotransmitters make a postsynaptic cell harder to excite. This is accomplished by hyperpolarizing the membrane, making the inside of the postsynaptic cell more negative with respect to the outside, so that a greater subsequent depolarization is required to bring the membrane to threshold. This hyperpolarizing potential is termed an *inhibitory postsynaptic potential* (IPSP). Both EPSPs and IPSPs are graded potentials.

The postsynaptic cell, then, is bombarded by a continuing flow of neurotransmitters, some of which make the cell more likely to fire (that is, generate an action potential) and some of which make the cell less likely to fire. The result of this bombardment is a continually fluctuating transmembrane potential. However, when the postsynaptic cell's membrane potential reaches threshold, an action potential is produced in the cell and is conducted over the length of the cell in the manner previously described.

From these synaptic events several important observations can be made. First, impulses are normally conducted in the nervous system in only one direction. This occurs because action potentials are propagated from the axon hillock toward the terminals and because neurotransmitters are released only at axon terminals, not at the dendrites. Second, although the conducted impulse in a given neuron is "all or none," the potentials at the synapse are finely graded. Finally, it is at synapses that the integration of nervous control of behavior takes place. Excitatory and inhibitory inputs from multiple neurons converge to produce or inhibit activity in a given postsynaptic cell.

*Motor or end plate potentials.* Besides stimulating or inhibiting other neurons, nerve cells may release neurotransmitters onto muscle or gland cells, and thereby influence their action. In the case of striate muscle cells, an axon terminal supplies each muscle cell, arriving at a specialized structure called the *motor end plate.* There the neurotransmitter acetylcholine produces a reduction in the resting potential of the muscle cell (the end plate potential) that nearly always initiates a muscle action potential. In some smooth muscle, the transmitter (typically acetylcholine or norepinephrine) is released at several places along the terminal ends of the axon and diffuses over the muscle cells (Guyton & Hall, 1996). By analogous mechanisms, neuronal action potentials can produce glandular secretion.

*A simple reflex: The function of receptor, synaptic, and motor potentials.* The three actions of neurons—receptive, synaptic, and motor—are easily seen in the simple monosynaptic reflex arc shown in figure 2.8. In most striate muscles, there are receptors that respond to stretching by initi-

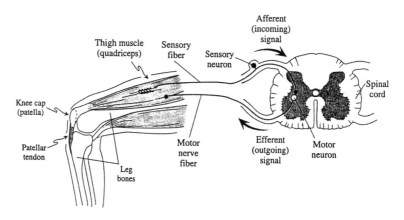

Figure 2.8. The monosynaptic reflex. The figure depicts the monosynaptic patellar tendon reflex. This reflex occurs when a tap on the patellar tendon stretches muscle fibers of the quadriceps muscle. The dendrites of a sensory neuron sense the stretch and pass this information to the cell body in the dorsal root ganglion (just outside the spinal cord) and then into the spinal cord. In the cord, there is a synapse between the axon terminals of the sensory neuron and the dendrites of the motor neuron. The signal travels across the synapse and initiates an action potential in the motor neuron, which results in contraction of the quadriceps muscle and an extension of the lower leg. Figure used with permission from G. G. Matthews, 1998, *Neurobiology: Molecules, cells, and systems*, Oxford, England: Blackwell Science.

ating action potentials in sensory neurons that terminate inside the spinal cord. At that synapse, a neurotransmitter is released which produces an EPSP in a motor neuron which in turn projects back to muscle fibers in the originating muscle. If the EPSP is of sufficient magnitude or if other excitatory impulses are arriving, action potentials will be initiated in the postsynaptic neuron. Once the impulse reaches the axon terminals, neurotransmitter will be released at the motor end plate and a muscle action potential will spread over the muscle, thus initiating movement.

## Bioelectric Potentials

The bioelectric events—both action potentials and the graded, synaptic potentials just described for neurons and muscles—provide an electrochemical record of neuromuscular functioning. By recording the appearance and passage of action potentials or graded potentials, the researcher can provide a representation of the action of nerves and muscles. By placing an appropriate electrode in or near a nerve or muscle cell and amplifying the observed potentials, the psychophysiologist records the activity of neural, muscle, and gland cells underneath the electrode. In general, the psychophysiologist's goal is to relate some aspect of behavior to the function of large systems of cells in the body which may be spread over a considerable area. For instance, we often record the electrical processes that initiate the beating of the heart (the *electrocardiogram* or EKG), the synchronous graded potential changes in millions of cortical brain cells (the *electroencephalogram*, EEG), or changes in the activity of many motor units in a muscle or muscle group (the *electromyogram*, or EMG). Moreover, as noted in chapter 1, the psychophysiologist, who usually works with human subjects, is typically restricted to recording these multicellular events from a relatively great distance, usually from the skin surface.

What are the relationships between cellular bioelectric events and the surface recorded potentials which are the primary interest of the psychophysiologist? In short, they are often difficult to determine. When action potentials or graded potentials occur simultaneously in a great number of cells, their summed potentials may be large enough to be recorded from the skin surface. However, the summed potential is difficult to relate to specific cellular functions; there are several reasons for this. First, cells that are nearer the recording electrode will contribute more to the recorded potential than those that are farther away. If, for example, a recording electrode is over a muscle, the motor units firing synchronously nearer the skin surface will contribute more to the surface EMG than motor units deep within the muscle tissue. Similarly, most of the activity recorded from the scalp as an EEG is the result of graded potentials arising from cortical brain cells rather than subcortical brain structures. Second, the orientation of cells firing action potentials can influence the appearance of a surface-recorded signal. Retreating action potentials (moving away from the electrode) will be seen as increasingly negative, whereas advancing potentials will be seen as increasingly positive. Repolarization also can produce measurable voltages at the skin surface. For instance, the T wave of the EKG is produced by the rapid repolarization of hundreds of muscle cells in the ventricles of the heart. Thus, a surface-recorded signal is a combination of potentials from many cells, some nearer the electrode, some further away, some which are moving toward the electrode and some away, some from cells which are depolarizing, others from cells that are repolarizing. The difficulties in interpreting such potential combinations is considerable.

Nevertheless, the potentials recorded from surface electrodes do result from underlying nerve and muscle action. Surface-recorded potentials result from either action potentials or graded potentials spreading over nerve or muscle cells and then through the body via the interstitial (extracellular) fluid that surrounds all cells of the body. Thus, very large signals such as those arising from depolarizing and repolarizing heart muscle which manifest as the surface EKG can be recorded between any two points on the body surface. However, the amplitude and waveform of the potentials spreading through the interstitial fluid are greatly changed as they spread. Like the ripple that forms in a pond into which a stone has been thrown, the potential becomes smaller as it spreads. In fact, the amplitude is so diminished that the waveform of the action potential from a single cell cannot be recorded from the surface of the skin. The amplitude of a signal is further reduced in passing through the high *impedance* of the skin. This is the reason that psychophysiologists recording a bioelectrical signal often must take great care to abrade the skin over which an electrode is to be placed. Abrading reduces the impedance of the skin to the passage of current between the tissue and the electrode. Recording principles such as the importance of abrading the skin will be discussed in greater detail where appropriate in chapters 7–13.

Despite the potential complications in interpretation, one can, by careful analysis and a knowledge of the underlying anatomy, relate surface-recorded signals to certain aspects of neuronal and muscular functioning. Thus, although there is not a simple mapping between the activity of a group of neurons and a signal on the skin's surface, knowledge about the underlying source of the signal recorded from the skin increases the likelihood that one can make appropriate inferences about the "meaning" of the signal. For example, during isometric contractions (where muscle tension is increased but muscle length does not change), EMG amplitude from electrodes placed over skeletal muscle fibers correlates reasonably well with the force generated, at least for moderate to high levels of contraction (Woods & Bigland-Ritchie, 1983). Likewise, the waves of the

EKG can be used to determine the timing of the electrical signal initiating cardiac contraction. The potentials with which the psychophysiologist works are, therefore, neither mysterious indices of cognitive or emotional function nor simple translations of physiological processes carried to the body surface. Rather, they are complex ramifications of the bioelectric spread of action potentials in a conductive medium, the human body.

### References

Berne, R. M., & Levy, M. N. (1998). *Physiology* (4th ed.). St. Louis, MO: Mosby.

Berntson, G. G., Cacioppo, J. T., & Quigley, K. S. (1991). Autonomic determinism: The modes of autonomic control, the doctrine of autonomic space and the laws of autonomic constraint. *Psychological Review 98*, 459–487.

Edwards, A. V. (1990). Autonomic control of endocrine pancreatic and adrenal function. In A. D. Loewy & K. M. Spyer (Eds.), *Central regulation of autonomic functions* (pp. 286–309). New York: Oxford University Press.

Gardner, E. (1975). *Fundamentals of neurology* (6th ed.). Philadelphia: Saunders.

Guyton, A. C. (1987). *Basic neuroscience: Anatomy and physiology*. Philadelphia: Saunders.

Guyton, A. C., & Hall, J. E. (1996). *Textbook of medical physiology* (9th ed.). Philadelphia: Saunders.

Ham, A. W. (1974). *Histology* (7th ed.). Philadelphia: Lippincott.

Loewy, A. D. (1990). Anatomy of the autonomic nervous system: An overview. In A. D. Loewy & K. M. Spyer (Eds.), *Central regulation of autonomic functions* (pp. 1–16). New York: Oxford University Press.

Matthews, G. G. (1998). *Neurobiology: Molecules, cells, and systems*. Oxford: Blackwell Science.

Morell, P., & Norton, W. T. (1980). Myelin. *Scientific American, 242*, 88–117.

Pansky, B., Allen, D. J., & Budd, G. C. (1988). *Review of neuroscience* (2nd ed.). New York: Macmillan.

Woods, J. J., & Bigland-Ritchie, B. (1983). Linear and non-linear surface EMG/force relationships in human muscles. *American Journal of Physical Medicine, 62*, 287–299.

# 3

# Equipment Used in
# Psychophysiological Recording

In chapter 2 we discussed the sources of the bioelectric potentials that can be recorded from the surface of the skin. The purpose of this chapter is to trace the bioelectric signals from the skin, across the junction with an electrode or transducer, into a polygraph or computer where it is filtered and amplified, and finally to the point where it is displayed and analyzed.

## Electrodes and Transducers

We will describe only those electrodes designed to be placed directly on the surface of the skin—cutaneous electrodes—although other types of electrodes exist (such as needle electrodes) for both human and animal work. In the second part of this section, we will discuss transducers for measuring temperature, respiration, and blood volume.

### Electrodes

Electrodes are usually small metal discs attached to the subject's skin for the purpose of recording the underlying electrical activity. Two electrodes must always be used and their location depends upon the particular physiological signal of interest. We discuss electrode location in the chapters dealing with specific measures. The one overriding concern in selecting electrodes and electrode paste and in preparing the skin is to provide a low-impedance, electrochemically stable path for the bioelectric potential from the skin to the input of the polygraph. The low impedance is necessary to keep the small bioelectric potentials from being seriously attenuated in crossing the skin, that is, before reaching the electrode. Chemical stability prevents the development of unstable potentials at the electrode, which would affect the biopotential. Electrodes are more than simply terminals or contact points from which voltages can be obtained on the surface of the body. Electrodes aid in converting ionic potentials generated by nerve, muscle, or gland cells within the body into electrical potentials that can be measured. Complications arise, however, when metals such as those commonly used for electrodes are placed in contact with an electrolytic substance, such as electrode paste or the skin. At the electrode-electrolyte interface, an electrochemical reaction is produced that creates a difference in voltage between the metal and the electrolytic solution. In this manner, voltages may be produced at the electrode site independent of the bioelectric event in the body. Thus, it is possible to record unwanted voltages produced at the electrodes in addition to the desired psychophysiological signal.

The potential or voltage produced by the electrodes themselves (the bias potential or offset potential, as it is referred to by some investigators) is a function of many factors, among them the particular metal, the type of electrolytic solution, and the temperature. In a historical study, Lykken (1959) constructed electrodes from different types of metals, placed them in pairs in a saline solution, and then measured the potential difference between the electrodes over time. After an hour, Lykken found that some metals showed greater potential difference than others. For example, he found platinum to produce a potential of 320 mV; silver, 94 mV; zinc, 100 mV; and chlorided silver (silver-silver chloride), only 2.5 mV. Thus, it is not difficult to understand why silver-silver chloride electrodes are preferred in most laboratories today. The advantage of silver-silver chloride electrodes is that (1) they introduce a relatively small initial measurement error (bias potential); (2) they show a relatively small drift of potential with use; and (3) they minimally develop polarization potentials.

With prolonged use, every pair of electrodes shows some polarization, the buildup of a counter-electromotive force, which has the effect of an apparent increase in subject resistance. Polarization can be thought of as the unequal distribution of ions on the two electrodes as a function of the passage of current through the electrolyte. That is, one electrode becomes positive in relation to the other, and the two electrodes therefore produce a potential or voltage of their own. Polarization generally can be reduced by leaving the electrodes connected together in a saline solution for several hours.

The electrodes in frequent use today are the floating or cup-shaped type that is seen in most research labs and a disposable version which is used by both labs and clinical settings. With this type of electrode, the metal part does not come in direct contact with the skin; it contacts the skin through a "cushion" of electrode paste. The floating or cup-shaped

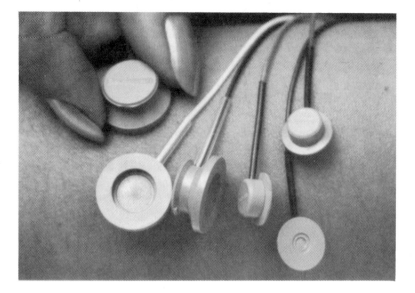

Figure 3.1. Commonly used floating or cup-shaped electrodes.

electrode (figure 3.1) is attached to the subject by an adhesive collar. The collar has an adhesive material on both sides that sticks to both the skin and the electrode, holding the electrode securely to the skin. Because of the jellylike consistency of the electrode paste, the floating electrode is less disturbed by small movements than electrodes rigidly affixed to the skin. Using these electrodes, it is even possible to record muscle potentials from moving athletes without significant artifact. Electrode paste is also used for two other reasons. First, it lowers the impedance between the electrode and the skin which is its most important function. Second, some types of electrode paste also help to stick the electrode to the skin.

An early study conducted by Lewes (1965) demonstrated that for some types of recording, many different electrode pastes will work satisfactorily. This study recorded the electrical activity of the heart using several types of electrode paste as well as no paste. In each case, the heart signal was as good as that recorded with standard electrode paste. What makes this interesting is that a standard laboratory electrode paste was compared with mayonnaise, French mustard, tomato paste, hand cream, and toothpaste! It should be noted that although almost anything works for heart rate recording, most of these substances probably will not suffice for signals of lower voltages, such as those recorded from muscles and the brain. Also, the excessive salt contained in most standard laboratory electrode pastes makes them unsuitable for recording some aspects of skin conductance and skin potential. In later chapters in this book dealing with individual physiological measures, we will emphasize when the characteristics of the electrode paste used are important. Although silver-silver chloride electrodes and improved electrode pastes have reduced many of the problems of recording, one must still be concerned about proper skin preparation in order to insure the best possible signal. Because the outer layer of the skin is mainly dead cells, dirt, and grease, these must be removed to lower impedance before the electrodes are applied. There are numerous methods for reducing skin impedance. One method is to abrade the area with fine sandpaper, an abrasive cloth, or an electrode paste which contains an abrasive material. The skin is then cleaned and dead cells wiped away with either alcohol or water. (This procedure must not be used when recording electrodermal activity; see chapter 13.) One should abrade the skin until it is somewhat reddish but not bloody. The report of an ad hoc committee of the Society for Psychophysiological Research (Putnam, Johnson, & Roth, 1992) offers guidelines for reducing the risk of disease transmission when applying electrodes to abraded skin. Once the electrodes are in place, resistance should be checked with an impedance meter. For a good recording, the impedance should be well below 10,000 $\Omega$.

The type of electrode and electrode paste used and the care that must be taken in skin preparation are a function of the signal to be recorded. Usually large amplitude signals can be satisfactorily recorded with minimal effort. However, weak signals or signals of low frequency require more stable electrodes and lower skin impedance. The greatest care must be taken when recording DC potentials, such as in skin potentials and certain brain potentials.

## Transducers

When energy changes form, it is said to be transduced. *Transducers* are used to convert physiological events to electrical potentials suitable for electronic amplification. All physiological responses must be transduced to voltage for the polygraph or computer even when the measure of interest is resistance or conductance. It is often convenient to record some result of nerve or muscle action rather than to record the action potentials themselves. For example, the pupil of the eye constricts and dilates through the contraction of muscle cells within the eye. While changes in pupil diameter are an interesting response, the muscle action potentials that produce them are difficult or nearly impossible to record directly. Alternatively, the result of the action potentials, the pupil diameter, may be more accessible and can be used to reflect underlying activity. If we transduced changes in pupil diameter to changes in some electrical parameter, those changes could be introduced to the physiological amplifier. In fact, we can use the amount of light reflected from the pupil onto a photosensitive resistor for the purpose. The possibilities for transducers are endless. Researchers can transduce any result of combined nerve, muscle, and glandular action to some form of electrical change. In practice, however, transducers typically respond to cardiovascular, respiratory, and somatic muscle changes with changes in their resistance to the passage of current. We will describe several of the more commonly used transducers here.

Most *strain gauge transducers* works on the principle that tension or strain in a metallic conductor changes the resistance and therefore the flow of electricity. A constant electrical voltage is applied to the metal, and changes in its resistance (due to changes in tension) are noted. One common application of the strain gauge is in the measurement of respiration. The specific type of gauge commonly utilized is a small, flexible tube filled with mercury which is placed in an extended position across the subject's chest or around the body. As the person inhales, the chest enlarges and increases the tension in the tube, thereby increasing the resistance in the circuit. In this manner, changes in resistance reflect respiratory movements (see chapter 10).

Another common transducer is the *photoconduction* cell (or photo cell), which varies its resistance with the amount of light that hits it. Researchers often use such cells to indicate changes in blood volume in some body area. Light in the red to infrared range passes through living tissue, such as the skin, but such light is poorly transmitted and readily reflected by blood. This principle is used to determine the amount of blood passing through a finger, toe, ear lobe, penis, or clitoris. A small light is focused on, for example, the finger and mounted next to the photo cell. As the blood enters the finger, the amount of light reflected back to the cell changes; thus one can observe a change in the resistance of the cell. This resistance change corresponds to changes in the amount of blood (see chapter 12).

A third type of transducer is a *thermoresistive transducer* or thermistor, a device that changes its resistance in relation to its temperature. One popular use of this transducer is the measurement of skin temperature, such as from the hand. As the temperature of the hand increases, the resistance of the thermistor changes.

## Polygraphs

*Polygraphs* record a physiological signal in a continuous analog fashion rather than digitally sampling it in discrete units as is the case with computers. Many psychophysiological laboratories employ a multichannel polygraph. Such devices can display one or many physiological events recorded on a paper chart. A polygraph generally has three separate components through which the signal passes before being displayed. The first is a coupler or signal conditioner, which is designed to make the electrical characteristics of all signals compatible, regardless of the type of transducer from which the signals originated. The second component is a preamplifier; the third is a main amplifier, which has the function of producing an output of sufficient voltage to drive the transcribing pens or standardize the voltage for computer storage and analysis.

### Couplers

The *coupler* conditions the psychophysiological signal coming from the subject. In some cases, the coupler does nothing more than supply the signal to the preamplifier; in other cases, the coupler changes the form of the signal to meet the requirements of the amplifier. Sometimes the coupler is used to provide external voltage to a transducer, electronic balancing, or calibration. Other couplers provide selective filtering or perform integration or rate computation. There are specialized couplers designed for heart rate, EMG, respiration, EEG, and other standard measures.

### Filtering

Filtering of the signal can occur in the coupler and/or in either the preamplifier or power amplifier. *Filters* remove or reduce (attenuate) certain parts of the input signal and allow other parts of the signal to pass. *Low-pass filters* allow only frequencies below a certain frequency to pass. For example, if a low-pass filter set at 12 Hz is introduced into a circuit, then all frequencies above 12 Hz would be attenuated or reduced. A *high-pass filter* is similar to a low-pass filter, except that it allows frequencies only above a certain frequency to pass unattenuated. A *notch filter* will attenuate only a small range of frequencies while allowing all others to pass undiminished. A notch filter may be described as a band-reject filter. Notch filters are most often set at 60 Hz (the frequency of AC current in the United States) or at 50 Hz (the frequency of current in Europe and other areas) to remove unwanted interference. Figure 3.2 shows a re-

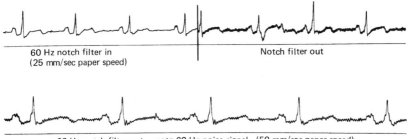

60 Hz notch filter in
(25 mm/sec paper speed)                    Notch filter out

60 Hz notch filter out — note 60 Hz noise signal   (50 mm/sec paper speed)

Figure 3.2. Recording of an EKG with and without a 60-Hz notch filter.

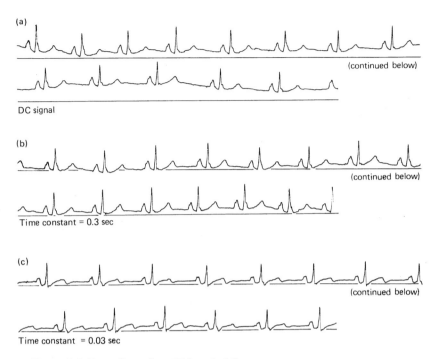

(a)

(continued below)

DC signal

(b)

(continued below)

Time constant = 0.3 sec

(c)

(continued below)

Time constant = 0.03 sec

Figure 3.3. Recording of an EKG with different time constants.

cording of an EKG with and without the 60-Hz notch filter. Another type of filter is the *band-pass filter*. This filter is really a combination of a high-pass and a low-pass filter adjusted such that only a certain range of frequencies can pass. For example, a researcher interested in the alpha rhythm (8–12 Hz) of the EEG, can set a band-pass filter to pass only those frequencies between 8 and 12 Hz and to attenuate all other frequencies.

Depending on how they are set, some couplers and amplifiers can handle either DC or AC signals. DC circuitry is designed for the recording of DC signals and signals of very low frequency. AC circuitry is designed for situations in which one wants to record higher frequencies and eliminate low frequencies. For example, EKG and EEG signals are generally recorded utilizing AC circuitry to avoid recording slow changes in potential, which would cause the signal to "drift" and thus make the changes of interest more difficult to interpret.

The reduction of the low frequencies in an AC circuit is determined by the time constant utilized. Stated simply, the time constant is defined as the amount of time required for a rectangular signal (step function) to return to 63% of its voltage. To illustrate this, figure 3.3 shows the same EKG recorded with different time constants. Note the difference in the baseline of the AC and DC recordings.

### Amplification

From the coupler the signal goes to the *preamplifier*, which increases the amplitude of the signal to a level that can be accepted by the power amplifier. The function of the amplifier is to increase the size of the physiological signal recorded at the surface of the skin to approximately 1 V. This typically will require an amplification factor or *gain* of at least 1,000. That is, a millivolt (1/1000 of a volt) would have to be amplified 1,000 times to equal 1 V. Since it is possible for nonphysiological signals (e.g., 60 Hz) to be picked up and amplified with the desired signal, there exists a term to describe the amount of signal (the biopotential) in relation to other electrical activity (generally referred to as noise). This is the *signal-to-noise ratio*. This ratio gives some indication of how much noise, or nondesired electrical activity, any electronic instrument will introduce. A term related to signal-to-noise ratio is common mode rejection. This refers to the amount of noise or interference present at the output of a differential amplifier. The higher the number in both cases, the better the physiological signal will be in relation to the noise of the total electronic environment in which the recording is taking place.

Today, the basic unit of construction for biomedical equipment such as amplifiers is the *integrated circuit* (IC). The integrated circuit is a multicomponent device (transistors, resistors, capacitors, diodes, and so forth) in which the components have been miniaturized and designed for specific purposes. For example, it is possible to purchase an inexpensive high-gain amplifier only a centimeter or so in size. An IC of this size may contain tens of thousands of components. Because of the IC, the psychophysiologist today is rarely required to construct complete circuits, or even to repair the existing ones, as was the case previously. However, it is important to have some knowledge of the types, properties, and functions of amplifiers, filters, and related coupling devices.

### Display

After the signal has been filtered and amplified, the power amplifier provides the voltage necessary to drive the recording device, usually a robust *galvanometer*. The galvanometer is an electromechanical device which uses a moving coil to drive the polygraph pen. Polygraphs can be purchased with ink-writing, heat-writing, or light-writing systems. Ink writing is the most common because the initial cost is less and the recording paper is considerably less expensive.

## Computers

The computer can be utilized to record and quantify data as long as the physiological signal can be converted into a numerical form. The device used to perform this function is the *analog-to-digital (A-D) converter*. The function of this device is to take a continuous signal and convert it into discrete steps. One way of thinking about an A-D converter is to imagine it as a voltmeter that samples at a very fast rate and then stores each of the samples. The speed at which the converter samples is referred to as the *sampling rate*. A good rule of thumb is that the sampling rate per second should be at least two to five times faster than the fastest frequency component of interest in the signal. This rule, the Nyquist relation, is discussed more fully in chapter 14.

Computers can also perform the functions described previously in terms of a polygraph, although they do this in a digital rather than analog manner. In terms of filtering, for example, the digital computer would use a mathematical formula rather than electronic circuitry to emphasize particular frequency components in a physiological signal. We will describe some of these mathematical transformations in the chapter on signal processing (chapter 14).

The computer also can be used to reduce the data. If the incoming signal is that of the biopotential from the heart and the desired measure is heart rate, then one does not need every value of the signal that is sampled. One would really only need to know when the biopotential was above a certain level, as in the case of the larger spike in the EKG, because this occurs precisely once per beat. A researcher could program the computer to compare each voltage coming from the A-D converter with a given voltage that was known to be present only when there was an EKG spike. A clock within the computer could be started and the time between each heart beat recorded and stored for future analysis.

A computer can also be utilized to recognize established psychophysiological patterns. For example, a researcher can program a computer to check a given EEG against a certain standard to determine if specific parameters are met. One example of such a use might be the determination of epileptic activity in the EEG. Or the computer might be used to determine whether certain frequencies, alpha for example, are present in the EEG signal. Using this type of analysis, the researcher could program a computer to give feedback or a type of stimulus only when certain preestablished conditions were met. For example, the presence of alpha activity without the presence of any eye movement could be one such combination. Although computers provide a means of making quick decisions concerning data, it must always be remembered that the computer makes its decisions in accordance with the instructions given to it. That is, a computer cannot discriminate any better than the person who programs it.

The ultimate value of the computer is that, if it is programmed properly, it can be designed to run entire experiments and even to analyze the data at the conclusion. This is particularly powerful in so-called real-time or *on-line* environments. For example, one could conduct a biofeedback experiment in real time; that is, the computer would provide feedback to the person in relation to actual physiological changes that were being made at that moment.

If data from an experiment were previously recorded on the computer disk or other storage device and the computer analyzed the data, the computer usage would be considered *off-line* and not in real time. That is, the experimenter could analyze the data in any manner or sequence desired without regard to how the events happened in real time. Let us end on one cautionary note. Although computers can quickly record and analyze physiological data, it is still critical that the researcher have a means for visually inspecting the data to determine that what is being recorded is an accurate physiological signal undistorted by, for example, movement, coughing, or electrical interference from other equipment.

*References*

Brown, C. C. (1967). *Methods in psychophysiology*. Baltimore, MD: Williams and Wilkins.

Cornsweet, T. M. (1963). *The design of electric circuits in the behavioral sciences*. New York: Wiley.

Cromwell, L., Arditti, M., Weibell, F. J., Pfeiffer, E. A., Steele, B., & Labok, J. (1976). *Medical instrumentation for health care*. Englewood Cliffs, NJ: Prentice-Hall.

Cromwell, L., Weibell, F. J., Pfeiffer, E. A., & Usselmann, L. B. (1973). *Biomedical instrumentation and measurements*. Englewood Cliffs, N. J.: Prentice-Hall.

Dewhurst, D. J. (1976). *An introduction to biomedical instrumentation*. Oxford: Pergamon.

Ferris, C. D. *Introduction to bioelectrodes*. (1974). New York: Plenum.

Geddes, L. A. (1972). *Electrodes and the measurement of bioelectric events*. New York: Wiley-Interscience.

Lewes, D. (1965). Electrode jelly in electrocardiography. *British Heart Journal, 27*, 105–115.

Lykken, D. T. (1959). Properties of electrodes used in electrodermal measurement. *Journal of Comparative and Physiological Psychology, 52*, 629–634.

Putnam, L. E., Johnson, R., & Roth, W. T. (1992). Guidelines for reducing the risks of disease transmission in the psychophysiology laboratory. *Psychophysiology, 29*, 127–141.

Venables, P. H., & Martin, L. (1967). *A manual of psychophysiological methods.* Amsterdam: North-Holland.

Welkowitz, W., & Deutsch, S. (1976). *Biomedical instruments. Theory and design.* New York: Academic Press.

Zucker, M. H. (1969). *Electronic circuits for the behavioral and biomedical sciences.* San Francisco: Freeman.

# 4

# Psychophysiological Recordings

... somatic responses abound. One has but to observe them on
a set of recording instruments to believe that they are by far the
most numerous responses of the organism. It is clear that any
overt response, vocal utterance, or bodily movement is surrounded
by a wide penumbra of them, and it may not be too bold a guess
to say that whenever there is any evidence of a stimulus affecting
the individual, something in his periphery or viscera is set into
motion. Not infrequently these may be seen when there is no
other means at hand for detecting that the person has been
stimulated.

(Davis, Buchwald, and Frankmann, 1955)

Somatic responses such as heart rate and muscle potentials do indeed
abound. Electrical activity can be recorded from the surface of the skin
at any moment. Background electrical activity is always present and
spontaneous changes in activity occasionally appear, even when it seems
that an individual is relaxing or asleep. This makes the task of recording
and correctly interpreting a subject's evoked response to a specific stimulus or situation a challenge.

Most psychophysiological recordings can be analyzed in terms of three
types of activity: *spontaneous, tonic* (background), and *phasic* (evoked responses).

Figure 4.1 shows a section of a typical recording. We will refer back
to this figure in this chapter as we define and discuss spontaneous, tonic,
and phasic activity.

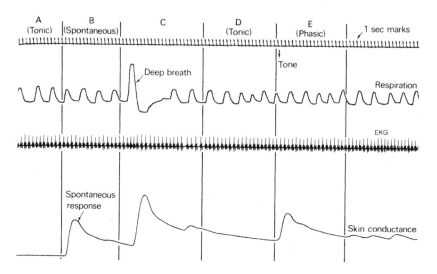

Figure 4.1. Recording of respiration, EKG, and skin conductance showing spontaneous, tonic, and phasic activity.

## Spontaneous Responses

What does a spontaneous physiological response to an unknown stimulus look like? It is the same as a physiological response to a known stimulus such as a tone, a shock, or a snake. It may take the form of a change in heart rate or skin conductance in the palm of the hand, muscle potential, and so on. Spontaneous activity is a name given in ignorance to what may be several different types of responses. What is referred to as spontaneous activity is in reality a change in physiological activity that occurs in the absence of any known stimuli.

Point B in Figure 4.1 shows an increase in heart rate and an increase in skin conductance to an unknown stimulus. In most if not all cases, such a spontaneous response would be the result of some CNS activity. For example, the subject might have just had an anxious thought about what procedure the experimenter was going to perform. However, unless the subject is asked about these thoughts immediately following the response, the experimenter would not know the cause of the so-called spontaneous activity. Changes in heart rate, skin conductance and/or other physiological responses that follow a deep breath, movement, or a cough—that is, following identifiable stimuli—are not considered to be spontaneous responses. Point C, in figure 4.1 shows such a series of events. Spontaneous ANS responses that involve no CNS activity have not been studied by psychophysiologists and probably occur rarely if at all. An example would be an increase in skin conductance that results from localized biochemical changes immediately under the recording electrode.

Why are spontaneous physiological responses of interest? When conducting research, it is important to be aware of the existence of such responses in order to avoid misinterpreting the data resulting from a study of the effects of some known stimulus on specific physiological activity. An obvious example would be the presentation of a stimulus to the subject while the subject is making a spontaneous response. The net effect might be a response greater than normal; then again, it might be smaller if the spontaneous response is in the opposite direction. In either case, quantification of the stimulus-contingent response will be difficult.

## Tonic Activity

Tonic activity is often referred to as the background level or resting level of activity of a particular physiological measure. However, resting level is not a good description of tonic activity because what we are really discussing is the level of activity when a subject is (1) not making a spontaneous response and (2) not making a discrete response to a known stimulus. The subject might be highly aroused and certainly not resting. For example, the tonic level of one individual's heart rate while waiting in a dentist's office prior to a root canal operation might be 130 beats per minute. Another subject in the same situation, perhaps someone not so bothered by dental work, might have a tonic level of heart rate of 80 beats per minute. Thus, tonic level is simply the level of activity of some ANS or CNS measure at a particular point in time prior to stimulation. In figure 4.1, point A or point D would be considered examples of tonic activity. Point A is just prior to a spontaneous response; point D precedes a response to a tone.

There are two separate reasons for recording and caring about tonic level. First, tonic level is of interest in its own right as a measure of the activity of the ANS or of muscles or brain when the subject is not responding to a specific stimulus. In such cases it is a complex result of many factors, including CNS reactions to environmental and internal stimuli, plus the delicate interplay between the sympathetic and parasympathetic branches of the ANS. People with essential hypertension and tension headaches are examples of individuals with extreme tonic levels of responding. Individuals with essential hypertension have high blood pressure due to elevated levels of sympathetic nervous system activity which keep their blood vessels in a highly contracted state. Muscle potential recordings from individuals who suffer from frequent tension headaches reveal that even when they are not experiencing headaches, the muscles of their head and/or neck show higher levels of activity than those of people who do not have tension headaches.

The second reason tonic level is of interest is that in some cases the size of a response to a specific stimulus depends upon the tonic level as measured immediately prior to the stimulus. For example, if one's heart rate is already close to the highest level that that person's heart can beat, it is unlikely that any stimulus will make it go much higher. This relationship is referred to as the *law of initial values*. This is a general principle of psychophysiology and will be discussed more fully in chapter 5.

The tonic level measured immediately prior to stimulation is referred to as the *baseline*, the level of activity against which we compare the phasic response to a stimulus. One important issue in psychophysiological recording is how long the baseline period should be. The answer is that it should be long enough to provide a stable prestimulus level and long enough to provide sufficient data for an appropriate analysis. On the other hand, it should be short enough so that the subject is neither bored nor anxious about the delay in instructions. For example, in recording the electrical activity that accompanies the contractions of the stomach (the electrogastrogram or EGG; see chapter 11), we find that the signal stabilizes in about 6 min. However, even if the EGG stabilized in 2–3 min, we would still need to record for a minimum of 4 min because that is the minimum length of time needed for the type of analysis used with EGG recording. Gerin, Pieper, and Pickering (1994) presented data showing that a 5-min baseline period is sufficient for cardiovascular recording. They also provide evidence that the baseline is not effected by the anticipation of a stressful task. In addition to the length of the baseline period, a second related issue is what the subject should be instructed to do during the baseline period. Most experimenters just tell the participants to sit quietly and relax. But not all subjects will or can follow those instructions. Jennings, Kamarck, Stewart, Eddy, and Johnson (1992) have suggested giving subjects a simple cognitive task that will create what they call a "vanilla baseline" and standardize the mental activity of all subjects during the baseline period.

Most psychophysiologists are less interested in tonic level than in responses to specific stimuli. The present authors, about 50 years after Schlosberg (1954), support his warning that this emphasis on stimulus-contingent responses (that is, phasic responses) and relative neglect of tonic levels is analogous to not seeing the forest for the trees.

## Phasic Activity

Phasic activity is a discrete response to a specific stimulus—an evoked response. Point E in figure 4.1 shows a phasic response to a tone. Phasic activity can be an increase or a decrease in either the frequency or amplitude of a response, or a more complex change in wave form or latency.

The most important factor to consider when quantifying phasic activity is that the subject's response to, for example, a slide of an American flag is not being made against a background of zero activity. The subject is constantly responding to internal as well as external stimuli—somatic responses abound. Two difficulties sometimes occur: (1) determining the magnitude of a subject's phasic response to a specific stimulus and separating it from other phasic responses and from spontaneous activity, and (2) attempting to introduce a correction factor for the magnitude of the phasic activity as a function of the preceding tonic activity, that is, the law of initial values. We address these issues in chapter 5 and where relevant in Part II, for example in chapter 13.

### References

Davis, R. C., Buchwald, A. M., & Frankmann, R. W. (1955). Autonomic and muscular responses and their relation to simple stimuli. *Psychological Monographs, 69* (Whole No. 405).

Gerin, W., Pieper, C., & Pickering, T. G. (1994). Anticipatory and residual effects of an active coping task on pre- and post-stress baselines. *Journal of Psychosomatic Research, 38,* 138–149.

Jennings, J. R., Kamarck, T., Stewart, C., Eddy, M., & Johnson, P. (1992). Alternate cardiovascular baseline assessment techniques: Vanilla or resting baseline. *Psychophysiology, 29,* 742–750.

Schlosberg, H. (1954). Three dimensions of emotion. *Psychological Review, 61,* 81–88.

# 5

# Some Basic Principles of Psychophysiology

The basic principles of psychophysiological recording are generalizations workers in this field have arrived at based on thousands of psychophysiological experiments. A familiarity with these principles will not only provide the reader with information about certain relationships between psychological and physiological variables but will also alert the reader to factors—other than the independent variable—that might influence the data collected in a psychophysiological experiment. Therefore, in this chapter we will discuss some basic relationships that are of interest in themselves but that sometimes make it difficult to see the effects of other variables being studied or to interpret the results properly. With an understanding of these generalizations, the reader should be better equipped to design new psychophysiological studies and to understand earlier publications.

## Arousal and Habituation

### Arousal

The concept of *arousal* is so basic to psychophysiology that we will discuss it first. New students of psychophysiology, when asked what specific problem they would like to study, often respond in one of the following two ways: (1) "I would like to record a physiological measure of arousal and determine the relationship of arousal to some behavior, such as problem solving," or (2) "I would like to record a physiological measure so that I can see how aroused participants will get when I show them slides of something gruesome, such as a car crash." These students are usually making two assumptions. First, they assume that arousal extends along an unidimensional continuum from deep sleep to high agitation. Second, they assume that one's position on the arousal continuum can be determined by measuring any one of several physiological variables, such as heart rate or skin conductance. Before we discuss why both assumptions are too simplistic, let us briefly relate them to the theories of some well-known investigators.

The concept of arousal or activation has its roots in Cannon's (1915) notion of the unified body preparing for fight or flight. Duffy (1957) extended this concept to include the intensity aspect of all behavior. As shown in figure 5.1, Duffy hypothesized an inverted U-shaped curve relating level of activation to performance. If our measure of performance is how fast our participants can run the 100-m dash and our measure of level of activation is their heart rate, we might well obtain an inverted U-shaped curve. Those who are too minimally aroused may start slowly, and those who are too highly aroused may commit false starts or suffer from a feeling of "spongy knees" which often accompanies stage fright. For a more detailed account of Duffy's theory, we refer the interested reader to her book *Activation and Behavior* (Duffy, 1962). Other early investigators who were interested in the relationship of arousal to behavior were Lindsley (1952) and Malmo (1959).

Let us examine some of Lacey's (1967) criticisms of activation theory. Lacey suggested that there are at least three different forms of arousal: cortical, autonomic, and behavioral. He pointed out that each is very complex, not a simple continuum. He presented evidence showing that

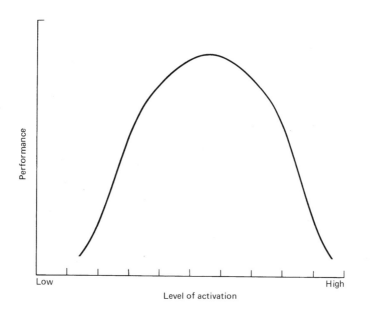

Figure 5.1. Duffy's hypothesized inverted U-shaped function relating level of activation and performance.

one form of arousal cannot always be used as a valid measure of another form of arousal. As an example of the complexities that exist within one form of arousal, consider autonomic indices of sexual arousal when heterosexual participants view slides of opposite-sex nudes. If we measure vasomotor activity in the finger, we would probably not detect any meaningful changes and might conclude that our participants are not aroused; however, if we record heart rate, we might come to a different conclusion. The explanation is that sexual arousal prior to climax is primarily a parasympathetic response, while vasomotor activity in the finger is governed by the sympathetic nervous system. Heart rate is controlled by both the parasympathetic and sympathetic systems; thus, we should expect to see some heart rate changes associated with the parasympathetic changes that accompany sexual excitement.

Another major criticism of activation theory can be found in the principle of *stimulus-response specificity*. Basically, this principle states that specific stimulus contexts—for example, noticing that your wallet or purse is missing—bring about certain patterns of responding, not just an increase or decrease in an unidimensional activation continuum. The pattern might include an increase in muscle tension, skin conductance, and respiratory amplitude, but a decrease in respiration rate and heart rate.

As a final point in his criticism of activation theory, Lacey referred to a special case of stimulus-response specificity which he termed directional fractionation. Picture the following scene and predict what is happening in terms of Lacey's three forms of arousal—cortical, autonomic, and behavioral. Four soldiers are in enemy territory, and it is late at night. One soldier is on guard duty while the others sleep. Suddenly there is an approaching noise in the darkness. What happens to the soldier's level of arousal? If we measure EEG activity, we would probably observe an increase in cortical arousal. If we measure skin conductance and heart rate as autonomic indices, however, we would likely find an increase in skin conductance, but a decrease in heart rate. This is what Lacey meant by directional fractionation—response directions are not uniform. Furthermore, if we observe the physical behavior, we would see that the soldier is probably standing very still, looking attentively toward the source of the noise and trying to determine if it is being made by friend or foe. A concept of activation based on a unidimensional continuum cannot deal adequately with such complexities.

## Habituation

The concept of *habituation* is just as basic to psychophysiology as the concept of arousal. In a sense, the two concepts are complementary.

Whereas arousal suggests heightened responding to a stimulus, habituation is the reduction of responding that occurs to the repeated presentation of the same stimulus. Habituation is a fascinating process to study in itself because of its ubiquity across a broad range of species and response systems; it is also important to be aware of habituation as an experimenter because it is commonly observed in psychophysiological experiments. For example, responses observed at the end of an experiment may be significantly smaller than those at the beginning because of habituation to the laboratory setting or to the repeated presentation of stimuli with similar features.

There are two general forms of habituation, short-term and long-term. Short-term habituation occurs within a single testing session. Figure 5.2 shows the short-term habituation of heart rate responses to a repeatedly presented 60 dB tone. Long-term habituation occurs when responses decrease in size over the course of multiple testing sessions separated by days or even weeks.

Numerous investigations have shown that responses generally habituate slowly to stimuli that are unique, complex, or intense. Responses habituate rapidly to stimuli that are presented frequently and slowly to stimuli that are infrequent. Habituation may be somewhat inhibited if the participant is required to make a behavioral response (e.g., to rate the subjective intensity of the stimuli) or if other stimuli—different from the repeated stimulus—are presented within an interstimulus interval.

Despite the wide range of species and responses that display habituation, there is no universally accepted explanation of why habituation

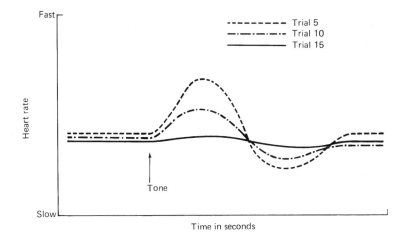

Figure 5.2. Habituation of the heart rate response to a moderate tone during trials 5, 10, and 15. Each data point represents the heart rate of one fictitious participant.

occurs. Among the most well-known theories of habituation are Sokolov's (1963) comparator theory of habituation and Groves and Thompson's (1970) dual-process theory of habituation.

Sokolov's comparator theory of habituation compares sensory information to a "neuronal model" of an anticipated stimulus. It was thought that the subject formed a model of a stimulus after the stimulus was presented many times. An assumption of the comparator theory was that when sensory input (i.e., a perceived stimulus) matches a model, a response to the input is inhibited. A mismatch between the input and the model was hypothesized to result in a response (e.g., orienting). The amplitude or strength of a given response was said to be a function of how well sensory input matches the model. Early in stimulus repetition, researchers observe strong responses because the mismatch between sensory input and the evolving model is large. After repetition, the model comes to represent the stimulus better; consequently, the mismatch between a stimulus and its model declines and response strength weakens.

Groves and Thompson proposed that two opposing processes—habituation and sensitization—simultaneously occur during the course of repeated stimulus presentation. According to Groves and Thompson, the habituation process mediates response decrement while sensitization acts to inflate response size. Habituation was thought to occur by decreased neuronal transmission along the stimulus-response pathway. Sensitization was thought to occur by increased activation of an organism's "state system," which governs general arousal. Groves and Thompson argued that a response incrementing process, such as sensitization, was a necessary postulate because increased—along with decreased—responding is commonly observed during the course of stimulus repetition, especially when the repeated stimulus is intense. For more information about how these two theories relate to the habituation of psychophysiological responses, see Graham (1973) and Stephenson and Siddle (1983).

## Orienting, Defensive, and Startle Responses

For more than seven decades, a considerable amount of research has been directed toward the study of *orienting, defensive,* and *startle responses.* The measurement of these responses has been utilized extensively in the study of development, emotion, learning, and attention in both humans and animals (see Campbell, Hayne, & Richardson, 1992, and Lang, Simons, & Balaban, 1997, for an overview). Because of the substantive role these responses play in the study of behavioral and cognitive processes, it is important to distinguish orienting, defensive, and startle response profiles. As an experimenter, it is also important to be aware of the types of stimuli that elicit these basic responses.

## Orienting Response

The orienting response directs our attention to novel stimuli and enhances sensory processing: it is the "what-is-it?" response. Beginning with Pavlov, Russian physiologists and psychologists studied this response extensively. Pavlov first became aware of the phenomenon when dogs, which had been conditioned by his students, failed to perform properly when he entered the laboratory. The problem was that the dogs paid attention to Pavlov—that, is they made an orienting response to him—instead of to the stimulus being presented by the student. Pavlov noted:

> It is this reflex which brings about the immediate response in men and animals to the slightest changes in the world around them, so that they immediately orientate their appropriate receptor organ in accordance with the perceptible quality in the agent bringing about the change, making a full investigation of it. The biological significance of this reflex is obvious. If the animal were not provided with such a reflex its life would hang at any moment by a thread. (1927, p. 12)

Some of the major components of the orienting response include (1) decreased irrelevant motor activity; (2) high-frequency, low-voltage EEG activity; (3) peripheral vasoconstriction and cephalic vasodilation; (4) increased skin conductance; (5) delayed respiration followed by an increase in amplitude and a decrease in frequency; and (6) heart rate deceleration (Graham, 1979; Graham & Clifton,1966; Lynn, 1966; Sokolov, 1963; Turpin, 1983, 1986). Note that peripheral vasoconstriction and cephalic vasodilation during orienting have been difficult to replicate and some authors have even reported that vasoconstriction in both the periphery and head occur to novel stimuli.

It appears that the function of this response is to prepare us to deal with novel stimuli—for example, the unexpected noise of an acorn falling on dry leaves while we are resting under an oak tree deep in the woods. Once we determine that the stimulus possesses no significance, there is no reason why we should prepare to deal with, for example, the noise made by other falling acorns. Because the orienting response is highly sensitive to stimulus novelty, it habituates rapidly after stimulus repetition (that is, after the stimulus becomes a common event).

## Defensive Response

Defensive responses are thought to protect us from the possible dangers of intense, painful, or threatening stimuli. Additionally, defensive responses trigger physiological adjustments that prepare an organism for action (e.g., "fight or flight"). These adjustments typically involve (1) increased skeletal muscle blood flow, (2) decreased blood flow to the gut,

(3) increased blood pressure, (4) peripheral and cephalic vasoconstriction, and (5) heart rate acceleration (Cannon, 1915; Sokolov, 1963; Turpin, 1979, 1983, 1986; Turpin & Siddle, 1978; Viken, Johnson, & Knutson, 1991). In general, defensive responses habituate slowly, but depending upon the intensity of a stimulus and the extent to which a repeated stimulus actually signals danger or induces pain, this response may habituate quite rapidly. In addition, Turpin (1986) suggested that homeostatic mechanisms may inhibit the repeated expression of a defensive response in a short time period.

### Startle Response

The startle response is elicited by an intense stimulus with a sudden or abrupt onset such as the crack of a lightening bolt. Graham (1992) contends that the function of the startle response is to interrupt or disengage an organism from ongoing activity. The human startle response involves both somatic and cardiovascular components. Using high-speed photography and the sudden shot of a pistol behind their participants, Landis and Hunt (1939) were among the first to note that the startle response involves a reflexive eyeblink and whole-body jerk. The startle response is also characterized by an immediate heart rate acceleration and rapid habituation of elicited physiological responses. Contemporary psychophysiologists employ stimuli of much less intensity than gunfire (e.g., short bursts of white noise) and typically focus on the eyeblink and heart rate components. It is important to note that components of the startle response differ from those of the defensive response primarily in speed. For example, the heart rate acceleration during startle typically peaks at approximately 4 s, whereas heart rate acceleration during a defensive response peaks at approximately 30 s (Reyes del Paso, Godoy, & Vila, 1993; Turpin, 1986). These differences are consistent with the functional importance attributed to each response; startle responses are thought of as fast acting and interruptive, but defensive responses involve more wide spread neurohumoral adjustments that facilitate behavioral action.

A practical reason for becoming aware of the circumstances under which orienting, defensive, and startle responses normally occur, and what they look like, is that the physiological response of participants to an independent variable in an experiment might be confounded by (that is, intermixed with) these responses. For example, whenever a series of slides is presented, the subject's responses to the first few will be partly caused by the content of those slides and partly by an orienting response. One way to deal with this problem is to disregard the data from the first few trials. Defensive or startle responses may be elicited during an experiment if participants hear a nearby door slam.

# Homeostasis and
# Autonomic Balance

## Homeostasis

The word *homeostasis* has been used to describe both a state of the organism and a process which takes place within the organism. When we refer to the homeostatic state, we are identifying equilibrium, stability, constancy, and the like. What we are really describing is a steady-state internal environment providing the right temperature, nourishment, oxygen, and fluids for optimal functioning of all cells. In our opinion, it is no more meaningful to specify the homeostatic state of the whole organism than it is to specify the stability of an entire city. In both cases, some parts (physiological systems or neighborhoods) may be very stable, while others are not. A typical statement appearing in the literature is: "Some animals are more successful than others in maintaining homeostasis." We feel that such a statement should always be qualified. In actuality, some animals are more successful in maintaining, for example, constant temperature, whereas others are more successful in maintaining constant blood pressure.

The mechanism that underlies the homeostatic process is negative feedback. However, the presence of the homeostatic state—that is, stability—is not invariably a sign of negative feedback. An example of a negative feedback system outside of our bodies is the thermostat that controls the temperature of a room. The thermostat senses the temperature; the warmer the room, the less heat it allows in.

Let us now examine Davis's (1958) analysis of the homeostatic control of body temperature in human beings. When we become too hot, regulation is accomplished by the evaporation of water secreted through the skin. Temperature is regulated, but what is happening to the sweating mechanism? Davis' answer was that every bit of reduced variation in temperature is brought about by increased variation in sweating. This he called *heterostasis*.

The general concept of homeostasis as first stated by Claude Bernard—"Le fixité du milieu interieur est la condition de la vie libre" ("The stability of the internal environment is the condition of a healthy life")—and later supported by Cannon (1939) in his book *The Wisdom of the Body* captured the imagination of physiologists and psychologists alike. The maintenance of equilibrium was accepted by some as the unifying principle of motivation and, indeed, as a model for many other aspects of behavior.

We believe that the following quotation from Davis (1958) puts the concept of homeostasis in better perspective: "Homeostasis exists, of course, with respect to certain variables, and one should try to find out what those are. But it is to be understood as a special case of the more general conception of the response of systems to inputs. There is no compulsion to think that the organism is an elaborate machine for the purpose of getting itself back to the status quo ante, or, indeed, for any other purpose" (p. 13).

Here is a practical example why the psychophysiologist should be aware of the possible complicating effects of homeostatic inputs. Stern (1976) studied heart-rate responses between the GET SET and GO of a race. In the initial design, subjects were instructed to get down on their hands in a typical sprinter's starting position, just prior to the GET SET. But the homeostatic response of the cardiovascular system to this postural change was a dramatic slowing of the heart. This effect was so great and long-lasting that it was not possible to determine the effect on heart rate of receiving the GET SET and waiting for the GO—the variable of interest in the study. To resolve this problem, in subsequent experiments subjects began from a standing position.

### Autonomic Balance

As mentioned in chapter 2, most internal organs, such as the heart, are innervated by both branches of the autonomic nervous system: the sympathetic nervous system (SNS) and the parasympathetic nervous system (PNS). The rate at which the heart beats is determined by the relative excitation from the SNS and PNS, or the autonomic balance. Autonomic balance may, therefore, be considered one specific part of homeostasis.

Eppinger and Hess (1915) were the first to classify people as *vagotonics* or *sympathicotonics*. Vagotonics (from vagus nerve, the primary parasympathetic nerve) are individuals who show unusually large responses to drugs that stimulate the PNS. Sympathicotonics are persons who show unusually large responses to drugs that stimulate the SNS. The interested reader is referred to early work on autonomic balance by Gellhorn, Cortell, and Feldman (1941) and Darrow (1943).

Wenger (1972) developed a technique for comparing an individual's resting scores on a group of ANS measures with the scores of other individuals and, in so doing, came up with an estimate of autonomic balance for each subject. Each score, called A, falls somewhere along a continuum, with low numbers indicating SNS dominance and high values indicating PNS dominance. For a given group of individuals, Wenger found that the scores are normally distributed; that is, few people—vagotonics and sympathicotonics—obtain extreme scores, and most fall in the middle. Wenger studied autonomic balance in children, college students, military personnel, and hospitalized groups. Interestingly, Wenger and his associates reported a higher incidence of psychosomatic, psychotic, neurotic, and physical disorders in people with low A scores.

## Modes of Autonomic Control

A more recent theoretical model of autonomic function (Berntson, Cacioppo, & Quigley, 1991, 1993) suggests that the sympathetic and parasympathetic nervous systems do not always act in an antagonistic or reciprocal fashion—that is, autonomic activity does not always fall somewhere along a continuum that extends from sympathetic to parasympathetic dominance. The major thesis of this model is that the two divisions can act independently, reciprocally, or even coactively (i.e., increase or decrease together). Furthermore, measures such as heart rate, which are influenced by both ANS divisions, provide little information about the specific mode of autonomic control underlying a given response. For instance, an increase in heart rate may be due to one of several possible patterns of autonomic activation: decreased parasympathetic activity, increased sympathetic activity, or even increased or decreased activity in both branches. In order to summarize all of the possible modes, Berntson et al. (1993, p. 297) advanced the bivariate representation of autonomic control shown in figure 5.3. The figure shows relative units of parasympathetic and sympathetic activity along the lower left and right axes of the model, respectively. The bidirectional arrows represent the possible modes of autonomic control over organs like the heart which receive both sympathetic and parasympathetic input. Arrows on the upper left and right axes represent the independent (uncorrelated) activities of the two autonomic divisions. The vertical arrow in the middle of the diagram represents a mode of coactivation, where activation of the two divisions may increase or decrease simultaneously. The intersecting horizontal arrow represents a reciprocal mode of control, where increased activity in one branch is accompanied by decreased activity in the other branch.

The mode of autonomic control that underlies a particular response is often determined by the selective pharmacological blockade of sympathetic or parasympathetic activity. In humans, this is particularly difficult, so many of the blockade studies that lend support to the model have been performed in nonhuman animals. For instance, Quigley and Berntson (1990) showed that heart rate deceleration to an orienting stimulus is no longer observed after parasympathetic blockade in the rat. This finding suggests that heart rate deceleration during an orienting response is mediated by increased parasympathetic activity; however, Quigley and Berntson also observed a notable acceleration to novel stimuli after parasympathetic blockade. This unexpected finding suggested that an orienting response may be mediated by an increase in the activity level of both autonomic divisions (i.e., coactivation), but the increase in parasympathetic activity—which is abolished after blockade—has a more powerful effect on the heart than does increased sympathetic activity. In this case, the increase in parasympathetic activity is said to mask the effects of the sympathetic division.

# Autonomic Space

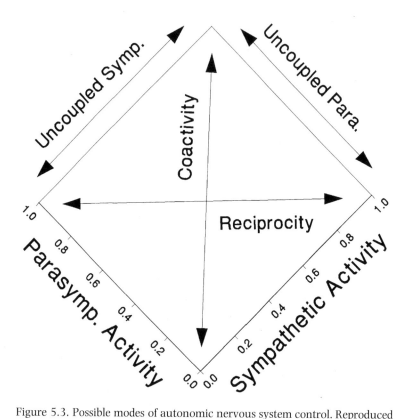

Figure 5.3. Possible modes of autonomic nervous system control. Reproduced with permission from G. G. Berntson, J. T. Cacioppo, & K. S. Quigley, 1993; "Cardiac psychophysiology and autonomic space in humans: Empirical perspectives and conceptual implications." *Psychological Bulletin, 114,* 296–322.

Noninvasive estimates of sympathetic (e.g., cardiac pre-ejection period) and parasympathetic (e.g., respiratory sinus arrhythmia) influences on cardiac activity have been well validated and are becoming increasingly employed in human research. We discuss these measures further in chapter 12.

## Law of Initial Values

In chapter 4, which dealt with tonic versus phasic measures of ANS activity, the *law of initial values* was briefly mentioned. In this section, we cover the relationship of the size of a response to the prestimulus level in greater detail.

Wilder (1967) was the first to call attention to this relationship and to name it the law of initial values (LIV). He stated that any increasing function would be smaller if the prestimulus level were higher and larger if the prestimulus level were lower. We would feel more comfortable with this formulation if Wilder had called it something like the principle of initial values. It is a principle that is often supported, but it does not hold at all prestimulus levels, for all subjects, or for all psychophysiological measures.

Before discussing when and where this principle does seem to hold, we must clarify what it conveys. Figure 5.4 shows fictitious data for the heart-rate (HR) response (increase in HR) to some stimulus as a function of prestimulus HR. Each data point represents the response of a different subject. This figure indicates that for these data, the magnitude of the increase in HR was strongly related to the prestimulus level. As would be predicted by the LIV, the greater the prestimulus level, the smaller the response to stimulation.

What physiological explanation is there for the LIV? Most psycho-physiologists believe that homeostasis (negative feedback) is responsible for the LIV. If we think of the various feedback mechanisms that set the functional limits for HR and other variables, then a subject whose pre-

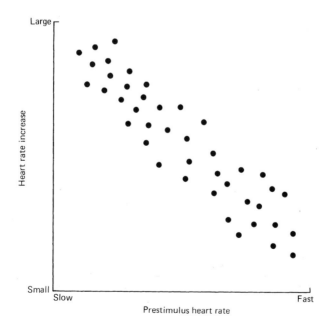

Figure 5.4. Heart rate response to a stimulus as a function of prestimulus heart rate. Each dot represents the heart rate for one fictitious participant.

stimulus level was 100 (subject B) was closer to the limit than a subject whose prestimulus level was 50 (subject A). Looking again at the function depicted in figure 5.4, which subject would be expected to show a greater increase in HR, A or B? We are now at the crux of the problem. Of course, subject A would be expected to show a greater absolute increase. But what about subject B? Shouldn't we inflate that subjects score, because stronger homeostatic mechanisms would have to be overcome due to a higher prestimulus level near the HR limit? Probably! Our answer would be a definite "yes" if there were sound evidence that it was more difficult—for example, took more metabolic energy—for subject B to go from an HR of 100 to 105 than for subject A to go from 50 to 65. Most psychophysiologists assume that this is the case, and the methods for dealing with the LIV discussed below are based on this assumption.

If we examine the evidence for the LIV from empirical studies, forgetting for the moment the previously mentioned assumption concerning the physiological basis, we find the following. For HR, most investigators have found that their results support the LIV. Most psychophysiologists have also found that skin resistance follows the LIV, but skin conductance usually does not. A few additional studies have found support for the LIV with blood pressure and respiration.

How would one know if a data set supported the LIV? An investigator could either calculate the correlation between the prestimulus levels and the magnitude of the response to stimulation, or could construct a scattergram such as figure 5.4. If a significant correlation does exist, how might we remove the effect of this relationship in further analyses?

Two methods are available for statistically neutralizing the LIV. Lacey's (1956) *Autonomic Lability Score* (ALS) is obtained from the following formula for each subject separately for each measure:

$$ALS = 50 + 10\frac{Y_z - X_z r_{xy}}{(1 - r^2 xy)^{0.5}}$$

In this formula, $X_z$ represents the individual's prestimulus level and $Y_z$ represents a poststimulus level, expressed in units of standard deviations from the total sample; $r_{xy}$ is the correlation for the sample between prestimulus and poststimulus levels. The constants 10 and 50 transform the resulting scores to a distribution with a mean of 50 and a standard deviation of 10. In other words, the ALS is a measure of the relative magnitude of a given subject's response compared to that which would be predicted from the linear regression between variables X and Y for the entire group. A score of 50 would indicate an average size response, 60 would indicate 1 standard deviation above the mean, and so on.

The second statistical method used to minimize the LIV is analysis of covariance (Benjamin, 1967). We will not describe in this book how to perform an analysis of covariance, but we will only make some general comments. Lacey's ALS is really a special case of the analysis of covariance. In the former, each individual's score is adjusted based on the correlation between group prestimulus and poststimulus scores. In the latter case, the group data are adjusted in much the same way so that the poststimulus scores of two groups that differed at prestimulus levels can be compared.

Comparing the size of responses of two subjects or two groups is very difficult. Lykken (1968) has suggested that we get a range of possible scores on each response measure of interest for each subject, then present the stimulus, and assign a score to each subject based on her/his minimum and maximum scores. Another possibility is to preselect subjects for two (or more) groups so that pairs of subjects have similar prestimulus levels.

This matter is so complex that when trying to write about it, we feel the way Cannon must have felt when Wilder wrote to him about the LIV. Cannon wrote back to Wilder that they were both too old to undertake the task. Cannon then was 68 years old, and Wilder was 44 (Wilder, 1967). Berntson et al. (1993), however, have recently attempted to relate the LIV to the model of autonomic control just described.

## Stimulus-Response Specificity and Individual Response Stereotypy

### Stimulus-Response Specificity

At the beginning of this chapter, we mentioned the concept of stimulus-response specificity, which makes a unidimensional activation continuum indefensible. The soldier standing guard duty at night who suddenly heard a noise displayed a specific pattern of responding which has been called directional fractionation. The soldier showed cortical arousal and an increase in skin conductance but a decrease in heart rate. Directional fractionation is a special case of stimulus-response specificity. What is germane to this discussion is that most other soldiers would have shown a similar pattern of responding in that stimulus situation. By definition, stimulus-response specificity exists if a stimulus brings about a similar pattern of physiological responding among most subjects.

Some investigators sought evidence of stimulus-response specificity to support William James's theory of emotion. James said that the perception of bodily changes is what constitutes emotion. Ax (1953) created a laboratory situation in which one group of subjects was made angry and another fearful. He recorded a large number of bodily responses and found that about half of them differentiated between the fear and anger situations. Davis (1957) sought response patterns to some simple stimuli with no notion of uncovering the physiological correlates of fear, repulsion, and the like. The various bodily responses recorded showed significant differentiation among the four stimulus situations: paced key pressing, listening to noises, looking at pictures, and receiving cutaneous stimulation. More recently, Stern and Koch (1996) showed that those subjects who report symptoms of motion sickness during illusory self-motion show a characteristic pattern of decreased respiratory sinus arrhythmia amplitude coupled with increased heart rate and gastric tachyarrhythmia.

## Individual Response Stereotypy

*Individual response stereotypy* refers to idiosyncratic responding. Will psychiatric patients who frequently complain of head and neck pain show a different pattern of bodily responses in a stress situation than patients who frequently complain of heart palpitation? That was the basic question asked by Malmo and Shagass (1949) in the first of a series of studies on what they came to call symptom specificity. They recorded heart rate changes, muscle potentials from the neck, and other physiological measures from both groups of patients. The exciting finding was that even when the stress consisted of only moderate thermal stimulation, and the subjects were not reporting that they were in pain, the head and neck complainers showed a significant increase in muscle potential from the neck, while the group that normally complained of palpitations showed a significant change in their heart rate.

Lacey and his co-workers conducted several studies during the 1950s (e.g., Lacey and Lacey, 1958) to see if the principle of symptom specificity would hold for nonpsychiatric patients. Using various groups of subjects and several different stressors, they found that individuals tend to respond by showing the greatest degree of activity in the same physiological system, no matter what the stress. For many subjects, their pattern of physiological responding was repeated from stressor to stressor. This is what we mean by individual response stereotypy.

Roessler and Engel (1977) made the point that stimulus-response specificity and individual response stereotypy are not mutually exclusive. For example, in the Davis (1957) study previously mentioned, the male subjects were shown a slide of a nude woman. Most, but not all, of the subjects displayed what Davis called the P pattern: increased skin conductance, peripheral vasoconstriction, and heart rate slowing. This would be an example of stimulus-response specificity. The fact that a few subjects responded differently, perhaps with a heart rate increase, may well be due to their idiosyncratic cardiac responding—another example of individual response stereotypy.

Stimulus-response specificity and individual response stereotypy probably exist to some degree in all psychophysiological studies. The practical question is, how serious is this problem, and what can and should be done about it? We cannot make a blanket statement concerning the proportion of the total variance in all future studies which will be attributable to stimulus-response specificity and individual response stereotypy, as it will no doubt vary considerably. However, the problem does not appear serious if careful consideration is given to the selection of physiological responses to be measured and the number of subjects. Stimulus-response specificity tells us that we should record not just one but several physiological measures and examine the pattern of responses to our various stimulus situations. Individual response stereotypy, on the other hand, alerts us to the problem of a few subjects making idiosyncratic responses in a situation where quite a different pattern of responses might be expected.

## References

Ax, A. F. (1953). The physiological differentiation between fear and anger in humans. *Psychosomatic Medicine, 15,* 433–442.

Benjamin, L. S. (1967) Facts and artifacts in using analysis of covariance to "undo" the law of initial values. *Psychophysiology, 4,* 187–206.

Berntson, G. G., Cacioppo, J. T., & Quigley, K. S. (1991). Autonomic determinism: The modes of autonomic control, the doctrine of autonomic space, and the laws of autonomic constraint. *Psychological Review, 98,* 459–487.

Berntson, G. G., Cacioppo, J. T., & Quigley, K. S. (1993). Cardiac psychophysiology and autonomic space in humans: Empirical perspectives and conceptual implications. *Psychological Bulletin, 114,* 296–322.

Campbell, B. A., Hayne, H., & Richardson, R. (Eds.). (1992). *Attention and information processing in infants and adults: Perspectives from human and animal research.* Hillsdale, NJ: Erlbaum.

Cannon, W. B. (1915). *Bodily changes in pain, hunger, fear, and rage.* New York: Appleton.

Cannon, W. B. (1939). *The wisdom of the body* (2nd ed.). New York: W. W. Norton.

Darrow, C. W. (1943). Physiological and clinical tests of autonomic function and autonomic balance. *Physiological Reviews, 23,* 1–36.

Davis, R. C. (1957). Response patterns. *Transactions of the New York Academy of Sciences, 19,* 731–739.

Davis, R. C. (1958). The domain of homeostasis. *Psychological Review, 65,* 8–13.

Duffy, E. (1957). The psychological significance of the concept of "arousal" or "activation." *Psychological Review, 64,* 265–275.

Duffy, E. (1962). *Activation and behavior.* New York: Wiley.

Eppinger, H., & Hess, L. (1915) *Vegatonia: Mental and nervous disease* (Monograph No. 20). New York: Nervous and Mental Disease Publishing Co.

Gellhorn, E., Cortell, L., and Feldman, S. (1941). The effect of emotion, sham rage, and hypothalamic stimulation on the vago-insulin system. *American Journal of Physiology, 133,* 532–541.

Graham, F. K. (1973). Habituation and distribution of responses innervated by the autonomic nervous system. In H. V. S. Peeke & M. Herz (Eds.), *Habituation. Vol. 1. Behavioral studies.* New York: Academic Press.

Graham, F. K. (1979). Distinguishing among orienting defense and startle reflexes. In H. D. Kimmel, E. H Van Olst, & J. F Orlebeke (Eds.), *The orienting reflex in humans* (pp. 137–168). Hillsdale, NJ: Erlbaum.

Graham, F. K. (1992). Attention: The heartbeat, the blink, and the brain. In B. A. Campbell, H. Hayne, & R. Richardson (Eds.), *Attention and information processing in infants and adults: Perspectives from human and animal research* (pp. 3–29). Hillsdale, NJ: Erlbaum.

Graham, F. K., & Clifton, R. K. (1966). Heart rate changes as a component of the orienting response. *Psychological Bulletin, 65,* 305–320.

Groves, P. M., & Thompson, R. F. (1970). Habituation: A dual-process theory. *Psychological Review, 77,* 419–450.

Lacey, J. I. (1956). The evaluation of autonomic responses: Towards a general solution. *Annals of the New York Academy of Science, 67,* 123–163.

Lacey, J. I. (1967). Somatic response patterning and stress: Some revisions of activation theory. In M. H. Appley & R. Trumbull (Eds.), *Psychological stress.* New York: Appleton Century Crofts.

Lacey, J. I., & Lacey, B. C. (1958). Verification and extension of the principle of autonomic response-stereotypy. *American Journal of Psychology, 71,* 50–73.

Landis, C. L., & Hunt, W. A. (1939). *The startle pattern.* New York: Farrar & Rinehart.

Lang, P. J., Simons, R. F., & Balaban, M. (Eds.). (1997). *Attention and orienting: Sensory and motivational processes.* Mahwah, NJ: Erlbaum.

Lindsley, D. B. (1952). Psychological phenomena and the electroencephalogram. *EEG and Clinical Neurophysiology, 4,* 443–456.

Lykken, D. (1968). Neurophysiology and psychophysiology in personality research. In E. F. Borgatta and W. W. Lambert (Eds.), *Handbook of personality theory and research.* Chicago: Rand McNally.

Lynn, R. (1966). *Attention, arousal, and the orientation reaction.* Oxford: Pergamon.

Malmo, R. B. (1959). Activation: A neuropsychological dimension. *Psychological Review, 66,* 367–386.

Malmo, R. B., & Shagass, C. (1949). Physiologic study of symptom neurosis in psychiatric patients under stress. *Psychosomatic Medicine, 11,* 25–29.

Pavlov, I. P. (1927). *Conditional reflexes. An investigation of the physiological activity of the cerebral cortex.* London: Oxford University Press.

Quigley, K. S., & Berntson, G. G. (1990). Autonomic origens of cardiac responses to nonsignal stimuli in the rat. *Behavioral Neuroscience, 104,* 751–762.

Reyes del Paso, G. A., Godoy, J., & Vila, J. (1993). Respiratory sinus arrhythmia as an index of parasympathetic control during the cardiac defense response. *Biological Psychology, 35,* 17–35.

Roessler, R., and Engel, B. T. (1977). The current status of the concepts of physiological response specificity and activation. In Z. S. Lipowski, D. R. Lipsitt, & P. C. Whybrow (Eds.), *Psychosomatic medicine.* New York: Oxford University Press.

Sokolov, E. N. (1963). *Perception and the conditioned reflex.* Oxford: Pergamon.

Stephenson, D., & Siddle, D. A. T. (1983). Theories of habituation. In D. A. T. Siddle (Ed.), *Orienting and habituation: Perspectives in human research* (pp. 183–236). Chichester, England: Wiley.

Stern, R. M. (1976). Reaction time and heart rate between the GET SET and GO of simulated races. *Psychophysiology, 13,* 149–154.

Stern, R. M., & Koch, K. L. (1996). Motion sickness and differential susceptibility. *Current Directions in Psychological Science, 5,* 115–120.

Turpin, G. (1979). A psychobiological approach to the differentiation of orienting and defense responses. In H. D. Kimmel, E. H Van Olst, & J. F Orlebeke (Eds.), *The orienting reflex in humans* (pp. 259–267). Hillsdale, NJ: Erlbaum.

Turpin, G. (1983). Unconditioned reflexes and the autonomic nervous system. In D. A. T. Siddle (Ed.), *Orienting and habituation: Perspectives in human research* (pp. 1–70). Chichester, England Wiley.

Turpin, G. (1986). Effects of stimulus intensity on autonomic responding: The problem of differentiating orienting and defensive reflexes. *Psychophysiology, 23,* 1–14.

Turpin, G., & Siddle, D. A. (1978). Cardiac and forearm plethysmographic responses to high intensity auditory stimuli. *Biological Psychology, 6,* 267–282.

Viken, R. J., Johnson, A. K., & Knutson, J. F. (1991). Blood pressure, heart rate, and regional resistance in behavioral defense. *Physiology and Behavior, 50,* 1097–1101.

Wenger, M. A. (1972). Autonomic balance. In N. S. Greenfield and R. A. Sternbach (Eds.), *Handbook of psychophysiology.* New York: Holt, Rinehart & Winston.

Wilder, J. (1967). *Stimulus and response: The law of initial value.* Bristol: Wright.

# 6

# Safety and Ethics in a
# Psychophysiology Laboratory

## Safety

While the laboratory electrical environment is probably at least as safe as the modern home and ordinarily poses little threat of shock, there are important implications for the treatment of the subject, particularly concerning grounding.

It is standard procedure in some labs to attach a ground lead to the subject when recording psychophysiological measures. The reason for the ground connection in these cases is not as protection for the subject, but rather to minimize unwanted electrical signals. If left "floating," or ungrounded, the subject acts as an antenna, picking up unwanted voltages from the air, much as a radio antenna picks up radio signals. These voltage variations, particularly 60 Hz, are then amplified and appear on the record, obscuring the desired biological signal. However, a ground lead may expose the subject to electrical hazard. If the subject is connected to ground through a low-impedance lead, then any device not at ground potential which touches the subject or which the subject touches, such as a lamp with an old two-prong plug and a short circuit, will cause a current to flow through the subject to ground. Furthermore, subjects seldom need to be grounded today to obtain artifact-free recordings. Modern differential amplifiers provide sufficient common mode rejection to reject, at the amplifier input, those transient signals the subject ground was meant to eliminate. Some older polygraphs, however, specify that a ground lead be attached for certain types of psychophysiological recording. We suggest that the experimenter carefully read the user manual for the instrument before deciding to use a subject ground.

If a piece of equipment is moved for repair and its ground is not reconnected properly, the case of that unit becomes a potential hazard. Therefore, ground connections should be routinely checked. If the laboratory is moved, it is important to check in the new facility that the third prong in wall sockets is, indeed, attached to the building ground. It quickly becomes obvious if your recorder is not receiving power, but it will not be obvious if it loses its ground connection.

## Additional Safety Principles

### Plans for Medical Emergency

There is always the possibility that a medical emergency will occur while a subject is under your care. The emergency may be related to the recording you are doing or independent of it. In any event, there should be a prepared course of action. The plan will vary depending on the location of laboratory. In a hospital, qualified persons and proper emergency equipment, as well as established emergency procedures, already exist. However, in an academic setting, emergency procedures are usually not so clear, but every laboratory must have a plan of action in case of an emergency. It is imperative that there be a first aid kit and a phone in the laboratory next to which there is a list of numbers to call in case of an emergency. We also recommend that laboratory personnel receive training in basic first aid and, if possible, cardiopulmonary resuscitation (CPR).

### Unusual Recordings

While recording, you may observe an EKG, EEG, or other psychophysiological response that appears abnormal. The EKG signal may be irregular, or missing a component. EEG records may appear to demonstrate "spike and dome" waves indicative of medical problems. The student psychophysiologist should not mention such apparent abnormalities to the subject. In most cases, the unusual recording is not indicative of a medical problem. Any suggestion to the subject that there may be something wrong with the subject's heart, brain, or other organ may seriously worry the subject for no reason. There are many reasons for unusual recordings; interpretation should be made by an expert. Such recordings should be shown to an instructor or other person responsible for the laboratory. This individual will make the interpretation, after consulting with a medical doctor if deemed necessary, and advise the subject when appropriate.

### The Use of Electric Shock on Human Subjects

It was formerly a common procedure to use electric shock as a noxious or arousing stimulus while recording psychophysiological data. More recently, electric shock has been less used, both because it is ethically questionable and because of the danger of serious injury. While a complete account of the potential circuits created through the subject by the introduction of shock is beyond the scope of this chapter, we feel that the dangers inherent in the use of electric shock are great enough to advise against its use where bioelectric potentials are being recorded simultaneously. Indeed, many of the "shockers" currently in the storerooms of psychology departments could not pass any reasonable test for electrical safety. Certainly any device that involves a 117 V AC supply—that is, one that plugs into a wall outlet—should not be used. Battery-powered shock generators are less dangerous, but they should be used only under direct supervision and with the greatest care. Electrodes, for example, should be placed close to one another and far from vital organs. Currents should never be passed through the body.

## Ethical Considerations

Before recording begins, the psychophysiologist must consider ethical questions related to his procedure. Does the procedure involve physical stress or even the threat of it? Could the recording result in anxiety, shame, guilt, or embarrassment? Is the subject's physical safety assured? Will all promises made to the subject be fulfilled? Is the subject to be fully informed about the procedure? Will information about the subject be confidential? Is coercion involved? The list of questions can go on and on, but the psychophysiologist must raise these questions and answer them.

While there may be a desire to absolve oneself of ethical responsibility by turning it over to others—the instructor, the "use of human subjects committee" (often referred to as institutional review board or IRB), or even the subject—responsibility must remain with the experimenter. What is more, psychophysiological recording, by its very nature raises ethical questions. For example, in EGG recording, should male experimenters apply electrodes to the skin over the abdomen of female subjects? We recommend gender matching when electrodes are applied so as to reduce any embarrassment or anxiety on the part of the subject. Some use of human subjects committees now require this. Ethical issues are also raised when, for example, recording blood pressure, the electroencephalogram, or electrodermal activity provides the experimenter or technician with information about the subject not known to others and probably not even to the subject. Also, as detailed earlier in the chapter, some discomfort and an element of danger are necessarily involved in recording.

What if the subject becomes frightened of the electrodes? Who is responsible? How did the situation come about? Is the equipment completely safe? How sure should one be of its safety before attaching it to another human being?

Ethical questions balance the rights of the subject with the possible benefits of the procedure. The rights of the subject include the right to privacy, the right to know what is to occur, freedom from physical danger, and freedom from fear, anger, embarrassment, or other behavioral disturbance. Benefits may include benefits to the experimenter (who may be learning a technique), benefits to the subject (in the case of an EMG relaxation procedure, for example), and benefits to society through an advance in scientific knowledge resulting from the experiment.

How can one evaluate the dangers inherent in doing psychophysiological research, and how can they be balanced with the possible benefits of recording? In the final analysis, each psychophysiologist must make his/her own ethical judgment. Scientists whose research involves human subjects have studied the ethics of working with human beings and have devised principles that will guide the psychophysiologist. The American Psychological Association (1992) has published an article entitled "Ethical Principles of Psychologists and Code of Conduct." The article deals with ethical standards for all aspects of the varied work of psychologists, but only the standards that relate directly to research are listed here. Where interpretation of the principles is not clear, the psychophysiologist should refer to the complete article, where the standards are presented in greater detail.

### The Ethical Standards

6.06 Planning Research.

(a) Psychologists design, conduct, and report research in accordance with recognized standards of scientific competence and ethical research.
(b) Psychologists plan their research so as to minimize the possibility that results will be misleading.
(c) In planning research, psychologists consider its ethical acceptability under the Ethics Code. If an ethical issue is unclear, psychologists seek to resolve the issue through consultation with institutional review boards, animal care and use committees, peer consultations, or other proper mechanisms.
(d) Psychologists take reasonable steps to implement appropriate protections for the rights and welfare of human participants, other persons affected by the research, and the welfare of animal subjects.

6.07 Responsibility.

(a) Psychologists conduct research competently and with due concern for the dignity and welfare of the participants.

(b) Psychologists are responsible for the ethical conduct of research conducted by them or by others under their supervision or control.

(c) Researchers and assistants are permitted to perform only those tasks for which they are appropriately trained and prepared.

(d) As part of the process of development and implementation of research projects, psychologists consult those with expertise concerning any special population under investigation or most likely to be affected.

6.08 Compliance With Law and Standards.

Psychologists plan and conduct research in a manner consistent with federal and state law and regulations, as well as professional standards governing the conduct of research, and particularly those standards governing research with human participants and animal subjects.

6.09 Institutional Approval.

Psychologists obtain from host institutions or organizations appropriate approval prior to conducting research, and they provide accurate information about their research proposals. They conduct the research in accordance with the approved research protocol.

6.10 Research Responsibilities.

Prior to conducting research (except research involving only anonymous surveys, naturalistic observations, or similar research), psychologists enter into an agreement with participants that clarifies the nature of the research and the responsibilities of each party.

6.11 Informed Consent to Research.

(a) Psychologists use language that is reasonably understandable to research participants in obtaining their appropriate informed consent (except as provided in Standard 6.12, Dispensing with Informed Consent). Such informed consent is appropriately documented.

(b) Using language that is reasonably understandable to participants, psychologists inform participants of the nature of the research; they inform participants that they are free to participate or to decline to participate or to withdraw from the research; they explain the foreseeable consequences of declining or withdrawing; they inform participants of significant factors that may be expected to influence their willingness to participate (such as risks, discomfort, adverse effects, or limitations on confidentiality, except as provided in Standard 6.15, Deception in Research); and they explain other aspects about which the prospective participants inquire.

(c) When psychologists conduct research with individuals such as students or subordinates, psychologists take special care to protect the prospective participants from adverse consequences of declining or withdrawing from participation.

(d) When research participation is a course requirement or opportunity for extra credit, the prospective participant is given the choice of equitable alternative activities.

(e) For persons who are legally incapable of giving informed consent, psychologists nevertheless (1) provide an appropriate explanation, (2) obtain the participant's assent, and (3) obtain appropriate permission from a legally authorized person, if such substitute consent is permitted by law.

6.12 Dispensing with Informed Consent.

Before determining that planned research (such as research involving only anonymous questionnaires, naturalistic observations, or certain kinds of archival research) does not require the informed consent of research participants, psychologists consider applicable regulations and institutional review board requirements, and they consult with colleagues as appropriate.

6.13 Informed Consent in Research Filming or Recording.

Psychologists obtain informed consent from research participants prior to filming or recording them in any form, unless the research involves simply naturalistic observations in public places and it is not anticipated that the recording will be used in a manner that could cause personal identification or harm.

6.14 Offering Inducements for Research Participants.

(a) In offering professional services as an inducement to obtain research participants, psychologists make clear the nature of the services, as well as the risks, obligations, and limitations.

(b) Psychologists do not offer excessive or inappropriate financial or other inducements to obtain research participants, particularly when it might tend to coerce participation.

6.15 Deception in Research.

(a) Psychologists do not conduct a study involving deception unless they have determined that the use of deceptive techniques is justified by the study's prospective scientific, educational, or applied value and that equally effective alternative procedures that do not use deception are not feasible.

(b) Psychologists never deceive research participants about significant aspects that would affect their willingness to participate, such as physical risks, discomfort, or unpleasant emotional experiences.

(c) Any other deception that is an integral feature of the design and conduct of an experiment must be explained to participants as early as is feasible, preferably at the conclusion of their participation, but no later than at the conclusion of the research. (See also Standard 6.18, Providing Participants with Information about the Study.)

6.16 Sharing and Utilizing Data.

Psychologists inform research participants of their anticipated sharing or further use of personally identifiable research data and of the possibility of unanticipated future uses.

6.17 Minimizing Invasiveness.

In conducting research, psychologists interfere with the participants or milieu from which data are collected only in a manner that is warranted by an appropriate research design and that is consistent with psychologists' roles as scientific investigators.

6.18 Providing Participants with Information about the Study.

(a) Psychologists provide a prompt opportunity for participants to obtain appropriate information about the nature, results, and conclusions of the research, and psychologists attempt to correct any misconceptions that participants may have.

(b) If scientific or humane values justify delaying or withholding this information, psychologists take reasonable measures to reduce the risk of harm.

6.19 Honoring Commitments.

Psychologists take reasonable measures to honor all commitments they have made to research participants.

### References

American Psychological Association (1992). Ethical principles of psychologists and code of conduct. American Psychologist, 47, 1597–1628. (Also available at www.APA.org). Copyright © 1992 by the American Psychological Association. Reprinted with permission.

# PART II

# Psychophysiology of Specific Organs and Systems

# 7

# Brain

*Electroencephalography and Imaging*

The presence of recognizable electrical rhythms of the brain has excited the curiosity and imagination of both professionals and laypeople alike. Psychophysiologists, neurologists, and science fiction writers have been intrigued by the presence of brain activity and the possibility of having an objective noninvasive marker that reflects underlying psychological processes. Some have taken these ideas to the extreme by suggesting that these measures can tell us what someone is thinking or feeling or even if they are telling the truth. Although it is not that simple, some researchers have begun to use brain activity to help physically disabled individuals to communicate, to move paralyzed limbs, or even to reduce seizure disorders. As discussed in this chapter, the understanding of cortical processes through various forms of brain imaging is a complex task. Scientists have come to appreciate the complicated relationship that exists between electrocortical measures and cognitive, emotional, and behavioral processes. There is a variety of techniques available to help us understand the functioning of the brain. We begin with the measurement of electrical activity recorded from the scalp, electroencephalography (EEG).

## Spontaneous EEGs

Electroencephalography is a technique for recording electrical activity from the scalp related to cortical activity. The EEG in humans was first described by Hans Berger in 1929. In his first set of papers, Berger sought to determine what activities were related to the EEG. As a good scientist, he first determined that EEG was actually related to brain activity and not other physiological activity. In order to do this he showed that EEG was not related to cerebral pulsations, cerebral blood flow, blood flow through scalp vessels, heart rate activity, muscle activity, eye movements or electrical properties of the skin. Berger took his studies beyond the physiological level and was one of the first to suggest that periodic fluctuations of the EEG might be related in humans to cognitive processes such as arousal, memory, and consciousness. Today, we carry on this work by using EEG measures to help us understand such processes as sleep, attention, emotion, and preparation for movement.

To record an EEG, electrical signals of only a few microvolts must be detected on the scalp. This can be accomplished by amplifying the differential between two electrodes, at least one of which is placed on the scalp. Since the signal must be amplified almost one million times, care must be taken that the resulting signal is indeed actual EEG and not artifact. Later in the chapter, we will discuss some possible artifacts, but for now let us examine the EEG. The rhythmic variations of the EEG are continually present at the surface of the scalp from well before birth to death. In fact, the absence of the EEG for 24 hr has been used as an indicator of "brain death." The various frequencies and distributions of specific patterns of the EEG wax and wane, providing the brain researcher and clinician with a constant record of the changing patterns of electrical activity of the brain. Some aspects of the EEG may appear almost random while other fluctuations appear periodic. We have a variety of signal-processing techniques to help us describe the EEG, but in general we use two basic parameters: amplitude (how large the signal is) and frequency (how fast the signal cycles). Some EEG patterns are extremely reliable and can be visually observed, as would have been required in the days before computer analysis. These patterns have been identified by Greek letters such as α (alpha), β (beta), and θ (theta).

*Alpha activity* can be seen in about three-fourths of all individuals when they are awake and relaxed. Asking these individuals to relax and close their eyes will result in recurring periods of several seconds in which the EEG consists of relatively large, rhythmic waves of about 8–12 Hz. This is the *alpha rhythm*, the presence of which has been related to relaxation and the lack of active cognitive processes. If someone who displays alpha activity is asked to perform cognitive activity such as solving an arithmetic problem in their head, alpha activity will no longer be present in the EEG. This is referred to as *alpha blocking*. Typically, with cognitive activity the alpha rhythm is replaced by high-frequency, low-amplitude EEG activity referred to as beta activity.

*Beta activity* occurs when one is alert. Traditionally, lower-voltage variations ranging from about 18 to 30 Hz have been referred to as beta and higher frequency lower-voltage variations ranging from about 30 to 70 Hz or higher as gamma. Recent work suggests that gamma activity is related to the brain's ability to integrate a variety of stimuli into a coherent whole. For example, Catherine Tallon-Baudry and her colleagues (1997) showed individuals pictures of a hidden Dalmatian dog which was difficult to see because of the black and white background. After training individuals to see the dog, there were differences in the gamma band response suggesting differential responses to meaningful versus nonmeaningful stimuli.

Additional patterns of spontaneous EEG activity include delta activity (0.5–4 Hz), theta activity (5–7 Hz), and lambda and K-complex waves and sleep spindles, which are not defined solely in terms of frequency.

*Theta activity* refers to EEG activity in the 4–8 Hz range. Walter (1953), who introduced the term theta rhythm, suggested that theta was seen at the cessation of a pleasurable activity. More recent research has theta associated with such processes as hypnagogic imagery, REM (rapid eye movement) sleep, problem solving, attention, and hypnosis. In a review of theta activity, Schacter (1977) suggested that there are actually two different types of theta activity. First there is theta activity associated with low levels of alertness as would be seen as one falls asleep. Second, there is theta activity associated with attention and active and efficient processing of cognitive and perceptual tasks. This is consistent with the suggestion of Vogel, Broverman, and Klaiber (1968) that there are two types of behavioral inhibition, one associated with a gross inactivation of an entire excitatory process resulting in less active behavioral states and one associated with selective inactivity as seen in overlearned processes.

*Delta activity* is low frequency (0.5–4 Hz) associated with sleep in healthy humans as well as with pathological conditions such as brain tumors. This is also the predominant frequency of human infants during the first two years of life. Figure 7.1 displays some commonly observed EEG waveforms.

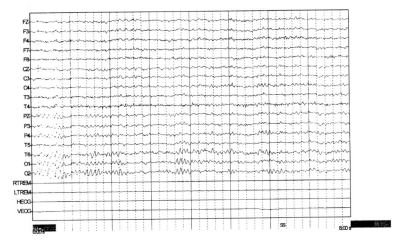

Figure 7.1. An EEG from an adult with electrodes at various sites on the scalp.

## Recording Procedure

Although procedures for recording EEG activity have improved greatly over the past 20 years with the incorporation of computer-controlled and digital amplifiers, one must still carefully consider how EEG is recorded and the possible artifacts that can compromise the data. Because EEG voltages are minuscule (several millionths of a volt) and thus must be amplified by a factor of a million, the possibility of recording electrical interference looms at every stage of instrumentation from the electrodes through to the recorder. These potentials can easily be confused with the legitimate EEG. Specific problems will be described in the appropriate sections of this chapter.

*Electrodes and Electrode Placement*   Where the electrodes are placed and how many are used depend on the purpose of the recording. Today, almost all EEG procedures use a variety of EEG helmets with up to 256 electrodes built into the helmet, although it is also still possible to record EEG from only two electrodes. Those recording helmets that use 128 to 256 electrodes are generally referred to as dense array EEG recordings. If the spatial distribution of some aspect of the EEG is the research question, then multiple electrodes distributed over the scalp are required. Of course, one can record from many fewer electrodes depending upon the empirical questions that are being asked. For example, if one is only interested in EEG responses associated with movement, then one may chose to record from regions of the scalp lying above the motor areas of the brain.

Historically, the system of locating electrodes in EEG is referred to as the International 10–20 system shown in figure 7.2 (Jasper, 1958). The name 10–20 refers to the fact that electrodes in this system are placed at sites 10% and 20% from four anatomical landmarks. In the front the nasion (the bridge of the nose) is used. In the rear of the head, the inion (the bump at the back of the head just above the neck) is used. The left and right landmarks are the preauricular points (depressions in front of the ears above the cheekbone). In this system, the letters refer to areas of the brain; O = occipital, P = parietal, C = central, F = frontal, and T = temporal. Numerical subscripts indicate laterality (odd numbers left, even right) and degree of displacement from the midline (subscripted z). Thus, $C_3$ describes an electrode over the central region of the brain on the left side, whereas $C_z$ would refer to an electrode placed at the top of the scalp above the central area. These lead locations are simply conventional and you may see in the literature nonstandard electrode location that are used in order to examine a particular research question.

Two specific types of EEG recording are called monopolar and bipolar recordings. In order to understand this point we must remember that

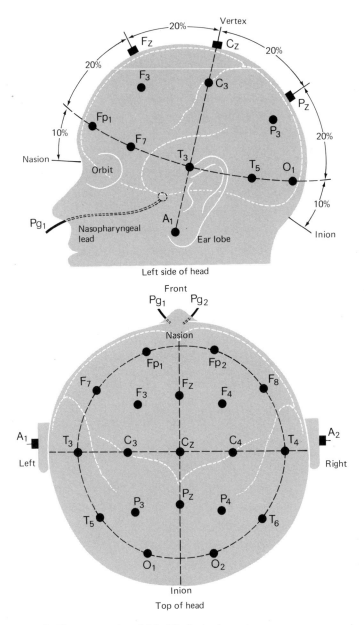

Figure 7.2. The international 10–20 electrode system.

EEG recordings reflect the difference in voltage between a signal at two electrodes. This means that if the exact cortical signal were present at two separate sites on which our electrodes were placed then we would record a straight line reflecting no difference in activity between the two sites. Of course, this never happens because there are always differences in activity between recording sites. In monopolar recordings the idea is to find a site that is not reflective of EEG activity per se to use as a reference site. Common sites used for this purpose are the ear (or ears), the mastoid, or even the nose. Both ears can be used as a reference site by connecting clip electrodes to each ear and then connecting these together as if they were one electrode. This technique is referred to as "linked ears." Thus, EEG activity from the various sites on the scalp could be referenced to the ear (or ears) to give the difference between each site and the reference electrode. Other researchers have suggested that a useful reference to use is that of the average reference. This procedure basically takes a network of electrodes spaced across the scalp and mathematically averages these together. This mathematical average value is then used as the reference.

In bipolar recording, each electrode is located to record from an active site on the scalp. Thus, one could compare the difference in EEG activity between the right frontal area with that of the left frontal area. One might use such a procedure to infer whether, for example, the left or right hemisphere was more involved in a particular task. This type of procedure has traditionally been used in clinical settings to identify unusual pathological waveforms, such as epileptic discharges.

*Recording Equipment*   Several types of *signal-conditioning* and amplification equipment may be used. Large hospitals and research laboratories employ multiple-channel electroencephalographs designed expressly for EEG recording. Many research labs also utilize a paperless EEG system which is controlled, displayed, and stored by the computer such that paper recording is not required. Psychophysiological laboratories may have one or more multipurpose polygraphs with signal-conditioning equipment that permits EEG recording. The amplifier used must have high gain capabilities and must be able to reproduce accurately the EEG signal at all desired frequencies. The amplifier must be able to amplify waveforms from almost DC (0 Hz) to more than 100 Hz. Typical amplification is a million or more times with little distortion. The amplifier must have an input impedance of several million ohms to prevent attenuation of the EEG signal. Also, the amplifier must have high common-mode rejection to reject ground-referred interference signals, such as 60-Hz interference from lights. Some systems may include a 60-Hz notch filter, which increases the ability to exclude interference of that frequency from the record, although distortion of waveforms at frequencies near 60 Hz may be introduced. It is helpful to have signal-conditioning filters that are used to emphasize a chosen range of EEG frequencies and to minimize others. Most commercial EEG recording systems include both high-pass and low-pass filters so that a "frequency window" can be constructed by setting the filters selectively to eliminate frequencies above and below those of interest. An important question we discuss in other chapters (see chapters 3 and 14) is the nature of a filter and what is referred to as roll off or sharpness. This simply asks the question of how does a 60-Hz filter, for example, affect nearby frequencies at 59 Hz and below and 61 Hz and above. Some systems describe the filters in terms of a time constant, which is basically the time it takes for an AC signal to fall two-thirds of its initial amplitude. According to the formula relating time constants and frequency, a time constant of 1 s, for example, attenuates all frequencies below 0.16 Hz, whereas a time constant of 0.03 would reduce signals below 5.3 Hz. Alternatively, a filter may be described in terms of the frequencies that are attenuated.

*Procedure*   As with most psychophysiological recording procedures, the basic requirement is to ensure that the areas under the EEG electrodes are free of hair, oils, and dead skin. If one were attaching a few electrodes, the areas to which electrodes will be attached are rubbed with alcohol or acetone to remove oils and dead skin. This should be done with care and patience, for the resistance between any electrode pair must be under 5,000 $\Omega$ to obtain a good recording. One may also slightly abrade the skin using a variety of procedures. An electrode paste (usually containing sodium chloride as the electrolyte) is rubbed into the skin at the electrode site. A similar procedure is used with electrode helmets in which as blunted needle is used to move the hair away from the electrode and a syringe like device used to inject electrode paste between the electrode and the scalp. It is imperative that the electrodes and the instruments used to prepare the scalp be disinfected between users to avoid spreading any pathogens. As mentioned in chapter 3, a committee of the Society for Psychophysiological Research developed a set of guidelines for the proper care and sterilization of EEG equipment (Putnam, Johnson, & Roth, 1992). Because of these concerns and with the development of dense array systems, a new technology is being developed that requires no skin abrasion prior to the application of EEG electrodes. Dense array systems use 128 or 256 electrodes; these new systems use a slightly different procedure because their amplifiers do not require lowering the impedance to 5,000 $\Omega$ as do the traditional systems. These systems are simply soaked in a solution and then applied directly to the head. Whether using these systems or the traditional methods, one must measure the quality of the connection, the impedance, between the scalp and the electrode. This measurement enables the researcher to ensure that all electrodes are functioning properly.

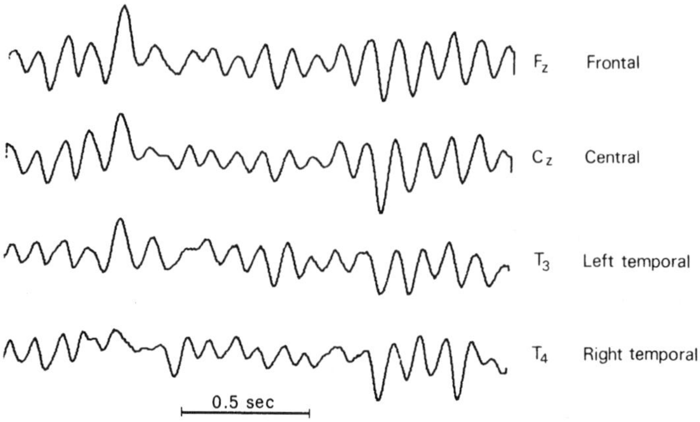

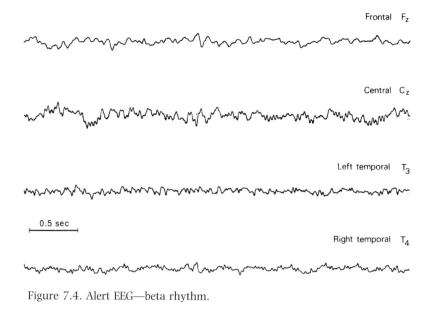

Figure 7.3. Resting EEG—alpha predominance.

## Typical Recordings

EEGs recorded under a variety of conditions are shown in figures 7.3, 7.4, and 7.5. Figure 7.3 shows four recordings obtained simultaneously from a resting subject. The four locations on the scalp from which the tracings were made are indicated in the figure: two temporal, one central, and one frontal. The high-amplitude waves seen in all the recordings are typical alpha rhythms. Figure 7.4 shows four recordings from the same scalp areas as in figure 7.3, but from an alert subject. Here we

Figure 7.4. Alert EEG—beta rhythm.

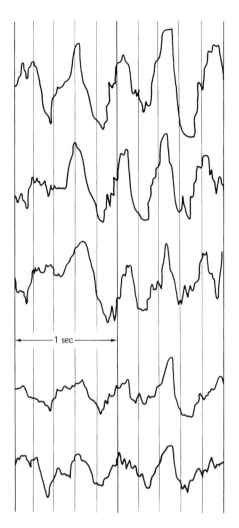

Figure 7.5. Delta waves recorded during deep sleep.

see typical low-amplitude fast waves—beta rhythms—along with some larger spikes. Sleep research is an area that makes much use of EEGs to determine if a subject is asleep and, if so, the stage of sleep. Figure 7.5 shows very the high-amplitude, very slow waves characteristic of delta rhythms. A record such as this would be obtained from a deeply sleeping subject.

### Common Problems

Given that the EEG signal is amplified more than a million times, *artifacts* can be a real problem in the EEG and misinterpreted as an actual signal.

For example, a student once interpreted an EEG to indicate a person was having an epileptic seizure when in fact the subject was chewing gum. Any type of movement can be seen in the EEG including muscle movement from facial expressions and talking. Another common artifact is related to eye movements which can interfere with the EEG signal. Today it is standard procedure when measuring the EEG to place electrodes around the eye to detect eye movement in any direction. These procedures are described in chapter 9. A variety of algorithms is available for removing eye movement signals from the EEG. The beating of the heart, which occurs at about once per second, also sometimes appears in an in a EEG record. External factors such as elevator motors or electric lights also can produce artifacts. Most of these problems can be dealt with by filters that reduce the unwanted frequencies. One of the best ways for students to learn about artifacts is to learn how to produce them on command. The presence of 60-Hz noise in the record is the most common difficulty in EEG recording. Figure 7.6 shows a continuous EEG in which 60 Hz is present in the first section but has been removed from the second section. Usually 60 Hz is recognized by its invariant frequency and amplitude. However, when it is of low amplitude, the presence of 60 Hz interference is not always as clear as in the example. This interference is often difficult to eliminate, in spite of the high common-mode rejection of modern differential amplifiers and the use of 60-Hz notch filters, because the source of the interference may be hundreds of times as powerful as the EEG signal generators themselves. If 60-Hz interference persists, it must be dealt with, since it will either obliterate the EEG or at least confound its interpretation. One common source of 60-Hz interference is fluorescent light fixtures. They may simply be turned off. Also, the interference may emanate from stimulus devices such as slide projectors, tape recorders, computer monitors, electric motors, and nearby electrical transmission lines.

The equipment and the subject may be isolated from all electrical interference by being enclosed in a grounded metal shield, but this is usually not necessary with newer recording equipment. For EEG record-

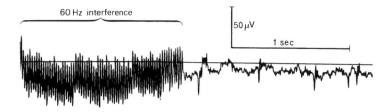

Figure 7.6. 60-Hz interference in an EEG record.

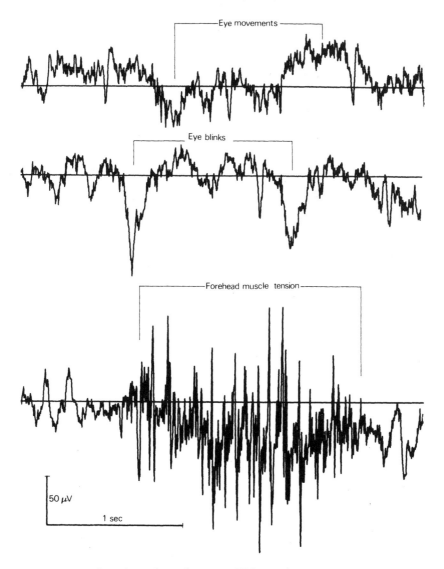

Figure 7.7. Physiological interference in EEG records.

ing, it is necessary that the subject be muscularly relaxed; head movements, jaw clenching, and frowning introduce large artifacts into the EEG. Subjects are usually instructed to fixate visually on some target or to close their eyes. Figure 7.7 demonstrates the effect of some of these physiological sources of interference on the spontaneous EEG. It is useful for the technician to be able to see the subject in order to identify better the source of artifacts.

## Analysis and Quantification

Historically, EEG technicians in clinical settings underwent extensive training so that they could recognize the visual patterns of EEG related to sleep stages and neurological disorders. Some frequencies, such as the alpha rhythm, are easy to recognize while detecting the presence of other EEG frequencies is more difficult. Since visual pattern recognition is subjective, EEG researchers have sought to develop quantitative procedures for describing EEG activity. In order to do a quantitative analysis, it is first necessary to convert the continuous analog EEG signal into a digital form, which is accomplished by an analog-to-digital converter. Once the signal is represented as individual numbers in a time series, these numbers can be manipulated mathematically. One of the first questions that must be determined is the sampling rate of the digital converter so that an accurate EEG record can be obtained. Based on a variety of engineering studies, the smallest sampling rate recommended is that of twice the highest frequency that one wishes to detect. Thus, if one wanted to study an EEG signal between 4 and 30 Hz, one would have to record the EEG at a sampling rate of at least 60 Hz. However, most researchers sample at four to eight times the highest frequency under consideration to ensure accurate detection of the EEG.

*Frequency Analysis*   One of the most common frequency analysis techniques is that of *Fourier analysis*. The technique is named after the French mathematician Fourier, who suggested that any given time series can be described as a corresponding sum of sine and cosine functions. Using this information he described how to determine in the frequency domain the amplitude and phase information of a known temporal signal. One simple way of understanding this procedure is to imagine that one had a variety of templates which represent each frequency band under consideration. Thus, one could have an 8-Hz template, a 9-Hz template, a 10-Hz template, and so forth. By simply placing each template on top of the signal, you could determine how closely the signal fit that template. This is basically the procedure that Fourier analysis uses. It takes an EEG signal over time and describes it in term of how much of each frequency is represented in the signal. Thus, Fourier converts a time-based signal to a frequency-based signal. In the 1960s a mathematical algorithm, referred to as the Fast Fourier Transform (FFT), was developed to speed computations of this procedure; FTT is used by most computer programs today. A more recent technique for frequency analysis, especially for short segments, is that of *wavelet analysis* (this is introduced in chapter 14).

An analysis technique related to Fourier analysis is that of coherence analysis. Whereas Fourier analysis gives the frequency for a given electrode, coherence gives the covariance of this measure for a pair of electrodes. Thus, coherence tells you how the EEG signal at each of two electrodes is related to each electrode. In simple terms, coherence reflects the manner in which two signals covary at a particular frequency. That is to say if the EEG at the right frontal electrode and the left frontal electrode both demonstrated a frequency of 8 Hz, then we would see greater coherence between the two electrodes than if they did not show the same frequency. In doing the coherence analysis, one can also obtain a measure of phase or synchrony. In other words, we can determine if two signals of the same frequency have peaks and valleys at the same time. Using coherence, Thatcher and his colleagues (1987, 1992) have studied how the brains of children develop patterns of EEG activity in different areas as they mature.

## Event-Related Potentials

### Evoked Responses

If a flash of light is viewed by a subject who has one electrode on the rear of his scalp and another on his earlobe, a predictable sequence of voltage variations will be recorded. A very small positive deflection (less than a microvolt) will follow the flash by about 40 ms. This response will be followed by a large negative deflection lasting 10 to 30 ms and peaking around 60 ms after the flash. Immediately following this wave there appears a fairly large, positive wave with a maximum amplitude occurring about 80 ms after the flash. This pattern is quite predictable; it follows each successive light flash, although, it should be stressed, with some variability from flash to flash. This succession of waveforms is termed the *visual evoked response*. When the distribution of the responses is examined, it is found to be of maximum amplitude over the occipital area of the brain, and to be less widely distributed than most spontaneous rhythms.

Other sensory-evoked responses also can be demonstrated. A sharp sound reliably produces an *auditory evoked response*. The response is maximal over the vertex of the brain and usually entirely absent from the occipital area. It has been shown that the brain's response to discrete sounds can be traced from the brain stem to the cortex in recordings from an electrode on the scalp. In such records (termed brain stem evoked responses, or BSERs), a distinct wave of positive voltage reflects each level of neural activity as the effects of the stimulus move through the brain. In the same manner, local stimulation of the skin surface in most body locations results in a somatic evoked potential, the waveform and distribution of which are dependent upon the area stimulated.

In general, evoked responses regardless of the nature of the stimulus are referred to as *event-related responses* (ERPs). Unlike the spontaneous

EEG, which is recorded in a continuous fashion over a period of time, ERPs are time locked to specific stimuli or responses. In the literature a distinction is sometimes made between endogenous and exogenous ERPs. Exogenous ERPs are seen to be controlled largely by the physical nature of the stimulus itself. Endogenous ERPs, on the other hand, are those that are influenced by the individual's perception or interpretation of the event. Most of the ERP research of interest to psychophysiologists would fall within the endogenous ERPs designation. Overall, the ERP is smaller in voltage than the EEG and requires averaging procedures over many trials for patterns to be clearly seen. The most common ERP procedure is to time lock the EEG signal to a particular tone or visual stimulus. By repeating the stimulus a number of times and averaging the electrocortical signal to each of these stimuli, it is possible to see a signal as displayed in figure 7.8. In this figure the stimulus presented at time 0 and the resulting ERP is seen to reflect the brain's processing of the information component of the stimulus. Traditionally ERPs are referred to in terms of whether the deflection is negative or positive and when the deflection occurs. Thus, a P300 component is a positive component occurring about 300 ms after the stimulus. It should be noted that the timing of

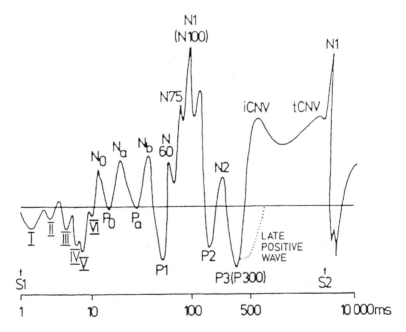

Figure 7.8. Averaged event-related response to acoustic stimuli. Waves I to VI comprise acoustic brain stem potentials. Components from 100 ms latency on are considered endogenous components. Reprinted with permission from B. Rockstroh, T. Elbert, A. Canavan, W. Lutzenberger, & N. Birbaumer, 1982, *Slow cortical potentials and behaviour*, Baltimore: Urban & Schwarzenberg.

the components are not precise but relative. While it is true that a P300 will follow an N200, the P300 may occur later than 300 ms. In viewing graphs of the ERP, a general procedure is to show the negative components as going upwards and the positive ones as downward. Unfortunately, this protocol is not always followed and one should carefully check the axes of a particular graph to determine how the ERP is plotted. To add to the confusion, ERP components may be abbreviated so that a N100 negative component may be referred to as N1, or a negative deflection that occurs approximately 200 ms after the stimulus referred to as N2.

In terms of time, the initial components of the ERP reflect automatic processing with the later components being more controlled and related to the cognitive processing of the stimulus. For example, if a pain stimulus was delivered to your right finger, an initial response would be seen on the left side of the cortex. At about 250 ms, an evoked response is seen that some researchers believe to be associated with the subjective response of pain. One of the most well known of the ERP components is that of P300, which in actuality can appear anywhere from 300 to 800 ms after the response. P300 is seen as reflecting cognitive processing and has been used in a variety of paradigms. For example, this component is larger if individuals are told to respond to a stimulus than if they are instructed to ignore it. One common P300 paradigm is that of the odd-ball. In this procedure, a series of tones with a similar frequency is played in which a tone of a different frequency is played randomly. The novel stimulus or "oddball" results in an increase in the amplitude of the P300. A related component involved with linguistic processing is that of the N400. This component seems to be especially related to linguistic expectation. For example, if you were to hear "Mary had a little . . ." you would probably expect the word "lamb" to come next. However, if you heard "Mary had a little pizza" then you would see an increase in the N400 component of an ERP.

## Slow Potentials

If you were told that after you heard a tone a picture would follow a few seconds later, you would notice a slow negative potential being generated once the tone sounded. This slow negative potential generally measured at the vertex is the *contingent negative variation* (CNV). The CNV is generated in the laboratory by presenting a first or warning stimulus which signals that a second stimulus will follow in a specific time period. In most studies the second stimulus signals cognitive or task processing. Walter (1967) described the CNV as an expectancy measure, because the first stimulus suggests that the second will follow.

Another form of event-related potential are very slow potentials that precede and accompany movement or other activities. If we ask a participant to press a button whenever desired, we discover that as early as a second before movement begins, a recognizable EEG waveform starts to develop. A recording made with an electrode placed over the central areas of the cortex displays increasingly negativity until, in the few milliseconds before a movement occurs, there is often a slight positive dip in the wave followed by a steep negative slope, which is terminated simultaneously with the beginning of the movement. The beginning of the movement is accompanied by a large positive deflection and a recovery to the original baseline. This complex of waveforms is not uniformly distributed. Technically, this slow increase in surface negativity is referred to as the *Bereitschaftspotential* (BP) or the *readiness potential* (RP).

The readiness potential is maximal at the vertex and initially equal in amplitude over both hemispheres of the brain. One research paradigm is to signal to the person which hand to use to make the movement. Prior to the movement, this potential begins to lateralize and becomes maximal over the motor cortex contralateral to the body part moved. Some researchers (e.g., Kutas and Donchin, 1980) have suggested that this beginning of lateralization reflects the point in time at which the response side is determined (i.e., to move the left or right hand). Since the information contained within the RP includes nonmotor processes as well as motor processes, researchers have suggested that by subtracting the response from one hemisphere from that of the opposite hemisphere, it would be possible to obtain a purer measure of motoric preparation for a response. This measure, referred to as the lateralized readiness potential (LRP), has become an important tool in the study of the neural basis of human cognitive-motor processing. Figure 7.9 illustrates the steps required to calculate the LRP.

To summarize, the development of this measure was based upon the assumption that the asymmetry of the RP could be used as an index for

Figure 7.9. Derivation of the lateralized readiness potential. The top panel shows idealized brain potentials from left $C_3$ and right $C_4$ scalp sites in a warned reaction time task, when subjects know in advance of the imperative stimulus the hand to be used to make a correct response. In the middle panel, potentials associated with left-hand movements are shown on the left; those associated with right-hand movements are shown on the right (WS=warning stimulus; IS=imperative stimulus). As subjects prepare to make a movement, a negativity develops that is maximum at scalp sites contralateral to the responding hand. The asymmetry in these potentials is illustrated by subtracting the potential recorded at the site ipsilateral to the movement from that recorded contralateral to the movement. Then the difference potentials for left-hand and right-hand movements are averaged to yield the lateralized readiness potential, bottom panel. Redrawn with permission from Coles, M. G. H., 1989, "Modern mind-brain reading: Psychophysiology, physiology, and cognition," *Psychophysiology, 216,* 251–269.

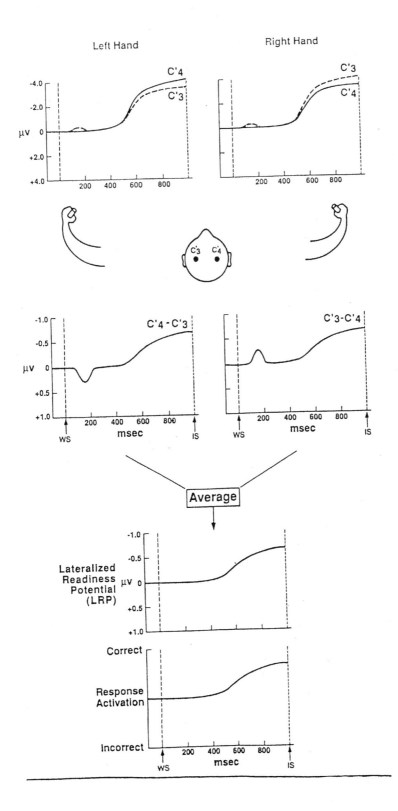

Left Hand

Right Hand

Average

Lateralized
Readiness
Potential
(LRP)

Correct

Response
Activation

Incorrect

the preparation of specific motor acts. To eliminate any RP asymmetries that may contain activity lateralized with respect to nonmotoric processes, the LRP was calculated as the difference between recording sites contralateral and ipsilateral to the responding hand, averaged over left- and right-hand responses (see de Jong, Wierda, Mulder, & Mulder, 1988; Gratton, Coles, Sirevaag, Eriksen, & Donchin, 1988, for alternative ways to calculate the LRP). The LRP's special significance in cognitive and sensorimotor research stems from the fact that this component offers a continuous analog measure of the differential engagement of the left hand versus right hand associated with cued or uncued voluntary reactions (see Hackley & Miller, 1995, for a review of this work).

The growing popularity of the LRP is due to the fact that its neuroanatomical and functional correlates are better understood than those of most other endogenous event-related potentials. Surface and depth recording indicate that the LRP is mainly generated by primary motor cortex. Moreover, the foreperiod LRP was found to be twice as large preceding complex movements (subjects were requested to press a sequence of three keys, using the index, ring, and middle fingers) than preceding simple ones (only index finger keystroke was required). Also, it has been reported that lateralization tends to be larger preceding a short sequence (one press with the index finger) than preceding a longer sequence (three presses with the same finger). These and other studies support the hypothesis that lateralized preparatory activity in motor cortex varies with specific properties of the planned movement.

The event related potentials, including evoked responses, the readiness potentials, and CNVs, are generally much smaller in amplitude than spontaneous EEGs and are therefore often not discernible in the raw or untreated record. In order to examine ERPs, special recording and data treatment procedures are necessary.

### Physiological Basis

What is the source of these recurring rhythmic potentials and event-related potentials? Until now, their definition and description have been entirely in terms of electrical comparisons between various points on the scalp surface and an earlobe, for example. But, what is under there? The brain, of course, with its more than 10 billion nerve cells, most of them synapsing with thousands of others. There are six layers of cells in the cortex which are referred to as layer I through layer VI. There are also other tissues in the brain. There are glial cells, whose functions are not yet entirely understood but which do generate a resting potential. There are also the fluids of the circulatory cerebrospinal system. The scalp itself, the skull, and the meninges covering the brain intervene between electrode and brain. However, the genesis of the EEG is clearly in brain tissue proper. Elul (1972) presented the arguments for this conclusion in careful and fascinating detail for those who would pursue the question. What structures actually produce EEG has been debated. One theory suggests that the EEG is generated by pyramidal cells in layers IV and V of the cortex.

Where a large group of cortical neurons is driven by identifiable volleys of afferent neural activity, as in the case of evoked potentials, the genesis of surface recorded waves is easily understood in terms of the mechanisms just described. But in the case of spontaneous rhythms, it is not at all obvious why the dendrites and synaptic connections of large groups of cortical neurons would vary in synchrony in a manner capable of producing the alpha rhythm, for example. While no firm answer can yet be given, it is probably that subcortical brain structures, particularly the thalamus, provide synchronizing signals to broad cortical areas. Brain stem mechanisms have also been shown to control some aspects of the EEG. Ascending discharges from the reticular formation cause a shift from alpha and slower rhythms to faster, less synchronized waves in cortical EEGs.

### Recording Procedure

*Electrodes*   Because some event-related potentials approach DC, the selection and preparation of electrodes must be undertaken with the greatest care. Otherwise, sizable slowly varying offset potentials may develop between electrodes, which can either obscure ERPs or confound their interpretation. Even with the best electrodes and most careful procedures, some drift often develops during ERP recording. Because silver-silver chloride electrodes are relatively nonpolarizing, are stable, and have a relatively low noise level, they are generally the electrodes of choice although gold, silver, or platinum discs have also been used for recording evoked potentials. Of all electrode types, the recessed pellets (composed of a compressed mixture of silver and silver chloride) are the most stable.

*Recording Equipment*   The amplifier must be capable of following voltages from DC to more than 100 Hz without distortion. It must have high input impedance and common-mode rejection capabilities equal to those required for recording the spontaneous EEG. Filtering and 60-Hz notch filters are useful but less vital to ERP recording than recording spontaneous EEGs.

*Averaging*   Some ERPs can be observed in a single trial before or after stimulation or responding, and some new techniques are being developed for single trial analysis. However, because ERPs are generally hidden in the spontaneous EEG, most techniques use signal-averaging procedures in which single trials are added together and averaged. ERPs are, by their nature, time-locked to known events, while spontaneous variations are not. If we compute an average of many repetitions of the event in which the event always occurs at the same point, then that portion of the EEG that regularly precedes or follows the event will remain in the average. The spontaneous variations will tend to cancel out over successive occurrences because a given wave is as likely to be positive as negative at any point in time. The result is a relative enhancement of the time-locked EEG, the ERP. A very rough representation of ERPs can be made by carefully measuring the amplitude of the EEG trace at several points which are time-locked to an event on 20 or more repetitive trials. The averages of these points can reveal the presence of an evoked or readiness potential. Today, this process is accomplished by a variety of computer programs.

*Procedure* The procedure for ERP recording is the same as that for recording spontaneous EEGs, but extra care should be given to electrode attachment.

## Typical Recordings

The effects of averaging are demonstrated in figure 7.10. In figure 7.10(a), EEGs for five single trials are compared to their average. The effect of increasing the number of trials on the averaged EEG is shown in figure 7.10(b). Figure 7.11 shows a comparison of somatic, auditory, and visual evoked potentials. Two types of slow potentials sometimes seen in the EEG are shown in figure 7.12. Figure 7.12(a) depicts the readiness potential (RP) and figure 7.12(b) the contingent negative variation, (CNV).

## Common Problems

Because ERPs are so small (1–10 µV), it is possible for an artifact occurring on a single trial to influence the appearance of the average. Additionally, time-linked artifacts may occur and be emphasized by averaging. In visually evoked responses, eye blinks may follow the visual stimulus on several trials with approximately the same latency. To preclude eye-blink effects in ERPs, electrodes are often placed near the orbit to monitor blinks and eye movements. Then, either the EEG record or the single trial record is examined for artifact, and only trials free from artifacts are included in the average.

## Analysis and Quantification

It should be recognized that considerable signal manipulation occurs in the averaging process. The averaged waveform is not necessarily a clearer version of that which occurs in each individual trial. In fact,

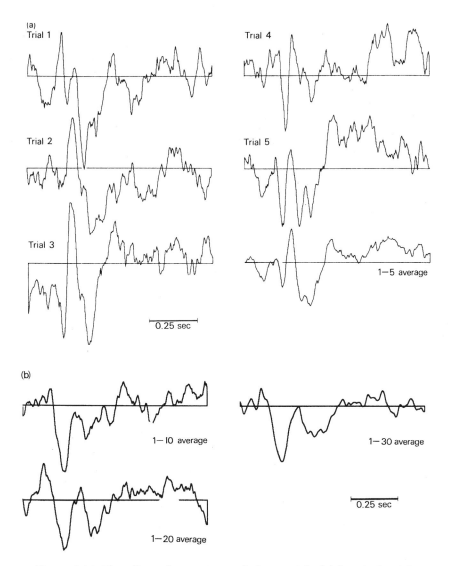

Figure 7.10. The effects of averaging evoked potentials: (a) five single trials compared to their average; (b) the effect of increasing the number of trials on the average.

differences between single trial ERPs might well be of interest but are lost in the averaging. Furthermore, ERPs do not occur with exactly the same latency from trial to trial, and this latency jitter will significantly influence the shape of the averaged ERP. Nevertheless, ERPs can be meaningfully subjected to numerical analysis.

To the degree that the waveform of an ERP is reliable, it can be compared to similar ERPs obtained under different circumstances. For in-

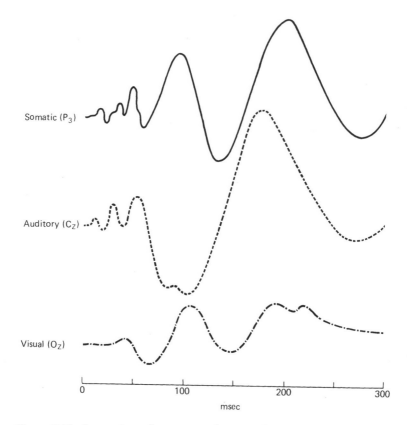

Figure 7.11. Comparison of somatic, auditory, and visual evoked potentials.

stance, the latency, or time from the event to specified points on the waveform, can be measured and compared in the usual statistical fashion. Amplitudes may also be measured at specified points relative to the event. The slope of an identifiable aspect of the wave and areas enclosed in waveforms can also be calculated. Figure 7.13(a) shows various possibilities for quantifying an idealized average evoked potential, while figure 7.13(b) demonstrates common approaches to quantifying slow potentials, the CNV and RP.

## Brain Imaging Techniques

EEG and ERPs have a real value in determining the time course of a response because they reflect millisecond changes within the electrical activity of the cortex. However, knowing where EEG activity takes place on the scalp does not in turn give you certainty concerning where the activity originated in the brain. This is referred to as the inverse problem.

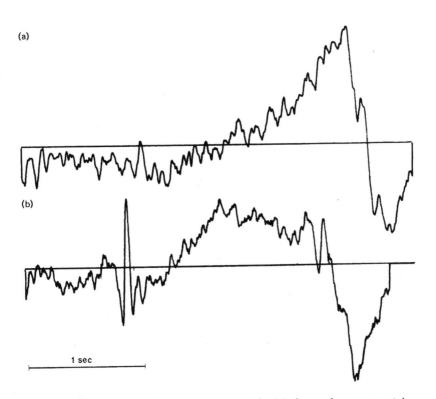

(a)

(b)

1 sec

Figure 7.12. Examples of slow wave potentials: (a) the readiness potential; (b) the contingent negative variation (CNV).

The problem reflects the fact that given a distribution of EEG activity on the scalp, there is a variety of possible distributions in the cortex that could lead to the same pattern of scalp activity. Other processes—such as the fact that electrical activity does not move uniformly through the brain and that there exists variation in the thickness of different individuals' skulls which influences how the brain's activity is distributed on the scalp—also add to the problem.

If you have ever placed a magnet under a piece of paper covered with iron filings, you know that by changing the position of the magnet you can change the pattern of filings on the paper. You can also do a similar procedure with electrical activity generated within the brain. Such a procedure is called dipole modeling. Using computers, one determines what type of pattern on the scalp would be produced by different generators in the brain. The pattern generated by the computer could then be compared to actual recorded EEG data. The computer can continue to move the dipole within the imagined brain until the theoretical pattern of EEG matches the actual pattern of EEG activity. Although dipole modeling offers one way of determining localization of activity, there are better

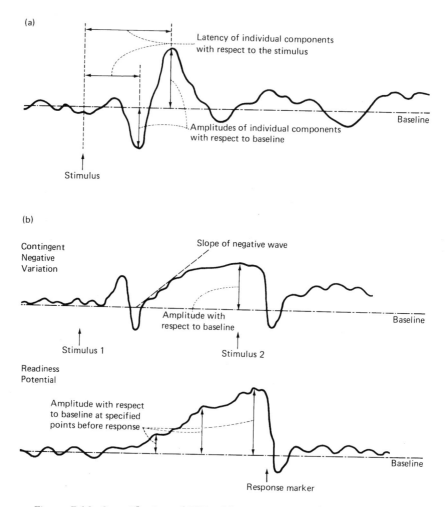

Figure 7.13. Quantification of ERPs: (a) measurement of evoked potentials; (b) measurement of contingent negative variation and a readiness potential.

methods for determining more exact localization of processes in the cortex. These are *magnetoencephalography* (MEG), *positron emission tomography* (PET), and *magnetic resonance imaging* (MRI).

Magnetoencephalography uses a SQUID (superconducting quantum interference device) to detect the small magnetic field gradients exiting and entering the surface of the head that are produced when neurons are active. MEG signals are similar to EEG ones but have one important advantage: magnetic fields are not distorted when they pass through the cortex and the skull, which makes localization of sources more accurate than EEG. It should be noted that MEG is only sensitive to tangential activity, which limits it to activity located in the sulci or cortical folds

In order to make a measurement, an individual simply places his or her head within the sensing device typically containing a large array of sensors that do not require physical contact with the head. Since measuring magnetic fields using MEG is a complex process requiring liquid helium (which must be supercooled 24 hr hours a day), the price of this system is expensive both to acquire and to maintain.

Positron emission tomography systems measure variations in cerebral blood flow that are correlated with brain activity. It is through blood flow that the brain obtains oxygen and glucose from which it gets its energy. By measuring changes in blood flow in different brain areas, it is possible to infer which areas of the brain are more or less active during particular tasks. Blood flow using PET is measured by injecting a tracer (a radioactive isotope) into the blood stream which is recorded by the PET scanner (a gamma ray detector). The general procedure is to make a measurement during a control task which is subtracted from the reading taken during an experimental task. Although it takes some time to make a PET reading (which reduces its value in terms of temporal resolution), the procedure is able to illustrate specific areas of the brain that are active during different types of processing. Since PET can measure almost any molecule that can be radioactively labeled, it can be used to answer specific questions about perfusion, metabolism, and neurotransmitter turnover. Some of PET's main disadvantages include expense, the need for a cyclotron to create radioactive agents, the injection of radioactive tracers (which limits the number of experimental sessions that can be run for a given individual), and limited temporal resolution.

Like PET, functional magnetic resonance imaging (fMRI) is based on the fact that blood flow increases in active areas of the cortex. However, it uses a different technology from PET; in fMRI local magnetic fields are measured in relation to an external magnet. Specifically, hemoglobin, which carries oxygen in the bloodstream, has different magnetic properties before and after oxygen is absorbed. Thus by measuring the ratio of hemoglobin with and without oxygen, the fMRI is able to map changes in cortical blood and infer neuronal activity. Although fMRI has the same temporal disadvantage as PET, it has a number of advantages including better spatial resolution and the ability to do repeated images on one individual.

*References*

Berger, H. (1929/1969). Über das Elektrekephalogramm des Menschen. *Archiv für Psychiatrie und Nervenkrankheiten, 40*, 527–570 reprinted in *Electroencephalography and Clinical Neurophysiology*, Supplement 28.

Buchsbaum, M., and Coppolar, R. (1974). Computer use in bioelectrical data collection and analysis. In R. F. Thompson and M. M. Patterson (Eds.), *Bioelectric recording techniques (Part B)*. New York: Academic Press.

Cole, M. G. H. (1989). Modern mind-brain reading: Psychophysiology, physiology, and cognition. *Psychophysiology, 26*, 251–269.

DeJong, R., Wierda, M., Mulder, G., & Mulder, L. (1988). Use of partial stimulus information in response processing. *Journal of Experimental Psychology: Human Perception and Performance, 14*, 682–692.

Donchin, E. (1961). Data analysis techniques in average evoked potential research. In E. Donchin and D. B. Lindsley (Eds.), *Average evoked potential: Methods, results, evaluations.* Washington, DC: National Aeronautics and Space Administration, NASA SP-191.

Elul, M. R. (1972). The genesis of the EEG. *International Review of Neurobiology, 15*, 227–272.

Glaser, E. M., and Ruchkin, D. S. (1976). *Principles of neurobiological signal analysis.* New York: Academic Press.

Gratton, G., Coles, M., Sirevaag, E., Eriksen, C. & Donchin, E. (1988) Pre- and poststimulus activation of response channels: A psychophysiological analysis. *Journal of Experimental Psychology: Human Perception & Performance, 14*, 331–344

Hackley, S., & Miller, J. (1995). Response complexity and precue interval effects on the lateralized readiness potential. *Psychophysiology, 32*, 230–241.

Jasper, H. H. (1958). The ten-twenty electrode system of the International Federation. *EEG Clinical Neurophysiology, 10*, 371–375.

Jewert, D. L., Romano, M. N., and Williston, J. S. (1970). Human auditory evoked potentials: Possible brain stem components detected on the scalp. *Science, 167*, 1517–1518.

Kutas, M., & Donchin, E. (1980). Preparation to respond as manifested by movement related brain potentials. *Brain Research, 202*, 95–115.

Lindsley, D. B. and Wicke, J. D. (1974). The electroencephalogram: Autonomous electrical activity in man and animals. In R. F. Thompson & M. M. Patterson (Eds.), *Bioelectric recording techniques (Part B).* New York: Academic Press.

Putnam, L. E., Johnson, R., Jr., & Roth, W. T. (1992). Guidelines for reducing the risk of disease transmission in the psychophysiology laboratory. *Psychophysiology, 29*, 127–141.

Rochstroh, B., Elbert, T., Canavan, A., Lutzenberger, W., & Birbaumer, N. (1982). *Slow cortical potentials and behavior.* Baltimore: Urban & Schwarzenber.

Schacter, D. L. (1977). EEG theta waves and psychological phenomena: A review and analysis. *Biological Psychology, 5*, 47–82.

Tallon-Baudry, C., Bertrand, O., Delpuech, C., & Pernier, J. (1997). Oscillatory gamma-band (30–70 Hz) activity induced by a visual search task in humans. *Journal of Neuroscience, 17*, 722–734.

Thatcher, R. W. (1992) Cyclic cortical reorganization during early childhood. *Brain and Cognition, 20*, 24–50.

Thatcher, R. W. Walker, R. A. & Giudice, S. (1987). Human cerebral hemispheres develop at different rates and ages. *Science, 236*, 1110–1113.

Vaughn, H. G. (1974). The analysis of scalp-recorded brain potentials. In R. F. Thompson & M. M. Patterson (Eds.), *Bioelectric recording techniques (Part B).* New York: Academic Press.

Vogel, W., Broverman, D. M., & Klaiber, E. L. (1968). EEG and mental abilities. *Electroencephalography and Clinical Neurophysiology, 24*, 166–175.

Walter, W. G. (1953). *The living brain.* New York: W. W. Norton.

Walter, G. (1967). Slow potential changes in the human brain associated with expectancy, decision, and intention. In W. Cobb and C. Morocutti (Eds.). *The evoked potentials. Electroencephalography and Clinical Neurophysiology,* Supplement 26, 123–130.

# 8

# Muscles

*Electromyography*

---

There are many reasons for recording muscle activity. Patterns of muscle action summate to produce movement and maintain posture; these patterns form the domain of kinesiologists and sports psychologists. Physical therapists record muscle action to document disabilities, to measure therapeutic progress, and to evaluate orthotic and prosthetic devices. The psychologist studying learning measures muscular activity in order to record the development of motor skills. The psychophysiologist, too, records muscle action, often when no movement occurs, as in the case of tension headaches or, more generally, to study the patterns of bodily reaction to stimulation, as in the startle response. One of the most significant uses of our muscles, as Darwin (1872) pointed out, is to communicate emotional expressions. Another use of muscles is to help us move quickly as when we are startled. Today, many psychophysiologists use the startle reflex as a way to measure emotionality. Let us examine this reflex in some detail.

The startle reflex, present in humans and other animals, is elicited by an intense stimulus of sudden onset which reaches maximum intensity in a short time. It has a short latency and occurs within 20 to 40 ms after the presentation of a 92 dB white noise burst in humans and other animals (Davis, 1984). The magnitude of the startle response can be decreased by presenting a less intense stimulus prior to the startle stimulus. This is called *pre-pulse inhibition*. Although less well studied, some stimuli (e.g., a light preceding the startle tone) have been shown to increase the startle response. This is called pre-pulse facilitation. An application of the prepulse work has been as a correlate of thought disorders in schizophrenics. In humans the startle reflex is often measured as the strength of the eye blink created by the orbicularis oculi muscle after an acoustic stimulus. We can measure many facets of the acoustic eye blink

106

startle reflex: these include blink magnitude, latency to blink, and habituation rate of blink response.

The startle response has been demonstrated in both humans and animals to reflect or result from reflexive modulation in relation to affective content (cf. Lang, 1995). The startle reflex also has been shown to be increased in magnitude during high (relative to low) arousal conditions (Vrana, Spence, & Lang, 1988) and during negative affective states such as fear, anger, and sadness relative to positive affective states such as joy and relaxation (Lang, 1995). Although the overall magnitude of the startle reflex decreases after repeated presentations of the startle stimulus, (i.e., the reflex shows habituation), the reflex continues to be stronger during negative relative to positive affect even after repeated presentations of the acoustic startle probe (Bradley, Lang, & Cuthbert, 1993). See figure 8.1 for an example of the startle reflex.

The question now arises about how to measure muscular activity. The means of recording muscle action range from filming whole body movements to the recording of action potentials from motor units within a single muscle. The choice of method should be made with careful regard for the aims of the procedure; each method has its particular virtues and shortcomings. Electromyography (EMG) is best suited for examining the way in which tension develops within a muscle, for determining the firing rates of particular motor units in relation to the recruitment of others, and for revealing activity too small to produce visible movement. But electromyography requires the attachment of electrodes, usually with accompanying wires that restrict movement. Furthermore, as will be detailed later in the chapter, EMG signals are subject to interference and distortion when movement occurs.

The EMG is a record over time of electrical potentials originating in muscles. EMGs may be obtained either by inserting electrodes into the muscle or by placing electrodes on the skin over the muscle or muscle group of interest. This chapter will describe only the techniques for the latter procedure, called surface electromyography. For a more in-depth

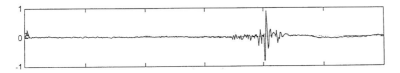

Figure 8.1. An example of the startle reflex. This figure shows an electromyogram (EMG) recorded from below the eye with the occurrence of a startle probe. In order to quantify the response, this signal would be rectified (all the negative values would be made positive) and integrated (the area under the curve would be computed).

discussion of the skeletomotor system, see Cacioppo, Tassinary, & Fridlund (1990).

## Physiological Basis

The cellular basis of EMGs is muscle action potentials spreading over skeletal muscle cells following neural stimulation. The intracellular result of muscle action potentials is contraction, as described in detail in chapter 2. A wave of depolarization can be recorded at a distance as a momentary difference in potential between electrodes spaced over the muscle. Since skeletal muscles are functionally divided into motor units which are activated in unison, action potentials are produced simultaneously in all the cells of a unit. The cells of a motor unit are usually distributed through a muscle rather than being concentrated at some point, and the firing of a motor unit produces a chord, so to speak, of action potential from the muscle. Seen from electrodes on the surface of the muscle, this chord will appear as a wave, the amplitude of which will be a function of the number of cells in the unit and their proximity to the electrode. Distant cells will contribute less to the wave than nearby cells will. If the interstitial fluid is considered to be homogeneous, then the contribution of a single action potential to the surface potential seen by an electrode will decrease as the square root of the distance from cell to electrode. Since the cells of the motor unit are usually dispersed longitudinally as well as radially, the sum of the individual cellular action potentials will differ in waveform from that of the single cells. The result is that the surface-recorded EMG resulting from the firing of a single motor unit will probably be unique, unlike that from other motor units within the muscle. When a skeletal muscle is nearly relaxed, the periodic firing of each of several motor units can be distinguished in terms of its amplitude, frequency, and waveform. In fact, in an early study Basmajian (1963), recording from needle electrodes inserted into the muscle, showed that voluntary control could be exercised over individual motor units. He reported that individuals were able to increase or decrease the rate of firing of single motor units.

However, as muscle activity increases, the time between action potential spikes becomes shorter and shorter as motor units increase their rate of firing. Other motor units are recruited until the firings of single motor units fuse with each other to produce a complex waveform that is no longer interpretable in terms of a motor unit.

More important for most applications, EMG can be related to the tension created in the muscle. In isometric contractions (when there is no movement), there is a close correspondence between the surface EMG summed over time and tension developed in the muscle over a wide range of tensions. However, the relationship does not hold for isotonic measurement, where movement occurs. This is partly because the tension developed in a muscle in response to a standard excitatory stimulus is a function of its length; in general, a muscle produces a smaller increment in tension at shorter initial lengths. Since a muscle becomes progressively shorter in an isotonic contraction, the length-tension relationship is continually changing. Also, as the muscle shortens, its fibers move under the electrodes, altering the relationship of the electrodes to the signal-generating tissue. Nevertheless, it has been determined that during constant velocity shortening there is a direct relationship between the integrated EMG and the tension exerted by the muscle.

The observed EMG varies from muscle to muscle, depending on the size of the muscle, the distribution of motor units within it, the size of the motor units, and the anatomy. Examples of typical recordings from various muscles are illustrated later in this chapter.

## Recording Procedure

Since the surface recorded EMG may vary in amplitude from a few microvolts to more than a millivolt, depending on the muscle and its state of contraction, the requirements for recording systems and procedures will vary with the intended use. If, for example, the aim of recording is simply to know when (or if) an arm or leg moved, the recording system need not be able to follow the tiny variations in tension which continually occur. A relatively simple system and somewhat crude procedures will suffice. However, to record the bursts attributable to single motor units, or to follow the buildup of tension before movement and when movement does occur, a system capable of high differential amplification must be used and accompanied by patient and careful recording procedures. The equipment and procedures described here are those for recording microvolt signals. The same equipment and procedures may be used for less sensitive recording, but with the amplifier sensitivity appropriately reduced.

### *Electrodes*

EMG electrodes should have the following characteristics: low impedance, low electrode potential (nonpolarizing), stability not subject to movement artifact, small size, and lightweight. If the electrode is either a combination of silver and silver chloride or carefully chlorided silver, it will be very stable, relatively nonpolarizing, and develop the smallest electrode potential of any available material. If, in addition, the electrode housing is constructed so that the electrode is of the floating, or liquid junction type—that is, the conductor is not directly in contact with the skin— then movement artifacts are greatly reduced. Floating silver-silver chloride electrodes are commercially available in several configurations (see chapter 3).

### Electrode Placement

The electrodes of a pair will record the difference in electrical potential between them originating in nearby, and to a lesser degree, distant muscle tissue. The placement of the pair and the distance between them, therefore, determines which muscles will contribute to the recorded EMG. The two principal considerations are: (1) both electrodes should be over the same muscle or muscle group, and (2) the pair should, where possible, be on a line parallel with the muscle fibers. A third factor, the distance between the electrodes of a pair, is dependent upon the length of the muscle and the desired discreteness of the EMG. Closely spaced electrodes (1 or 2 cm between them) will generally be superior for observing the activity of single motor units than a widely spaced pair, but not as good for obtaining an index of overall muscle tension.

In the case of the muscles moving the long bones of the skeleton, the application of these principles is relatively simple. For example, in order to record EMGs from biceps, the two leads, separated by 2 or 3 cm, are centered over the belly of the muscle (which may be located by palpation) in a line parallel with the underlying bone, that is, a line drawn from elbow to shoulder. If several recordings are to be made from the same subject, or if recordings from several subjects are to be compared, then care should be taken to identify the placements in terms of anatomical landmarks (see figure 8.2).

Since an electrode pair will record muscle potentials from nearby muscles, as well as the muscle under study, electrode placement and the interpretation of EMGs is difficult where several different muscles are near either electrode. Similarly, deep muscles may influence EMGs from electrodes over a superficial muscle.

In the forearm, the muscles moving the fingers, those bending the wrist, and those rotating the wrist are considerably interwoven. An EMG recorded from leads anywhere on the forearm will include, to some degree, contributions from all three muscles. A similar situation exists in the back, neck, head, and (to a lesser degree) the lower and upper leg. Electrode placement in these situations is arbitrary, and serviceable EMGs can be obtained by applying the principles just enumerated. There have, however, been attempts to standardize EMG lead placements. Some of

Figure 8.2. Atlas of EMG electrode placements. From J. T. Cacioppo and L. G. Tassinary (Eds.), 1990, *Principles of Psychophysiology*, New York: Cambridge University Press. Reprinted with the permission of Cambridge University Press.

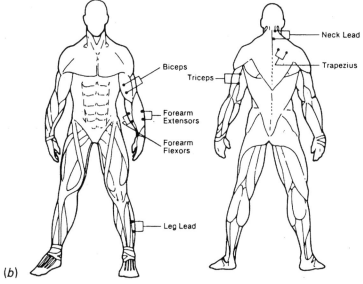

Ground

Lateral frontalis
Medial frontalis
Corrugator supercilii
Depressor supercilii/Procerus

Orbicularis oculi
(pars orbital)

Levator labii superioris

Orbicularis oris (inferior)
Depressor anguli oris
Mentalis

Zygomaticus major

Masseter

(a)

Biceps
Triceps

Forearm
Extensors

Forearm
Flexors

Neck Lead

Trapezius

Leg Lead

(b)

these are described by Cacioppo, Tassinary, & Fridlund (1990). Historically, Lippold (1967) includes descriptions of ten lead arrangements which were originally devised by J. F. Davis (1952). These placements, while they may be useful as guides, are arbitrary, and at least one of them (the forehead lead) violates the principles of electrode placement previously described (Davis, Brickett, Stern, & Kimball, 1978). That is, some individuals place frontalis electrodes horizontally across the forehead when in fact the muscles run in a vertical manner. We must reemphasize that regardless of the placement of electrodes, the EMG recorded from most locations will include contributions from other muscles. More will be said on this subject in the section on interpretation of EMGs.

### Recording Equipment

The requirements for amplification of EMGs are as follows: high gain, high input impedance, frequency response from 1 to 1,000 Hz. Since there is little or no DC in the EMG, capacitively coupled (AC) recording systems are preferred and selectively amplify fast voltage changes, thus ignoring steady states and very slow changes. Typical amplification systems include the clinical electromyograph, laboratory multipurpose polygraphs, and laboratory polygraphs with associated signal conditioning apparatus. Any of these systems is adequate if properly used. Since the frequencies in the EMG signal range up to 1,000 Hz, special consideration should be given to the frequency characteristics of the recording device. Most ink writing recorders are unable to follow reliably frequencies above 60 or 80 Hz. Thus, one should use an oscilloscope computer display for accurate portrayal of the signal. In using a computer system, it must be determined that the sampling frequency of the analog-to-digital conversion is sufficiently high to record the highest frequency components in the EMG.

Some EMG units, particularly those intended for biofeedback training, include no provision for displaying the raw, untreated EMG. Rather, their output is an auditory signal or visual (meter) display of the sum of the EMG. Such systems cannot be used for studying EMGs, although they may be useful for biofeedback training. Many EMG recorders include a provision for rectifying and, often, for integrating the signal as an addition or an alternative to direct recording. The function of integrators is described later in this chapter.

### Procedure

Electrode attachment must be accomplished with great care. After the electrode sites are chosen, carefully measured, and marked according to predetermined criteria, any hair under the site should be moved. The skin at the site is then cleaned with alcohol. Then the skin is abraded to remove the high-impedance dead surface layer of skin. The exposed area may be rubbed with electrode jelly, although the jelly will reduce the effectiveness of a electrode adhesive if it is allowed to spread beyond the central, active portion of the electrode. Also, any connection between the electrode paste or jelly at the sites of the two electrodes will reduce the recorded EMG. The electrodes must be firmly attached to the skin. Any movement of the electrodes will produce large artifacts.

The electrodes are prepared by coating or filling (in the case of recessed electrodes) them with electrode jelly. Some EMG electrodes are held in place by suction. Commercial electrodes that are affixed with collars with adhesive on both sides, are particularly convenient. Some laboratories employ a third, ground lead, for EMG recording, which is similarly attached. The impedance between the active leads of a channel should be tested with an impedance meter (preferably not an ohmmeter, because it will pass a DC current through the electrodes). The impedance of the pair should be 5,000 $\Omega$ or less. Higher electrode impedance will reduce the signal introduced to the amplifier and provide a possible source of interference. If the impedance is greater than 5,000 $\Omega$, the electrodes should be removed and reapplied after the underlying skin has been further abraded and new electrode jelly applied. The time spent in carefully applying electodes will be more than repaid by clear, interpretable EMGs later in the recording session.

The amplifier gain should be adjusted to the appropriate level for the type of recording to be generated. If single motor unit reponses or other low-level signals are of interest, then the gain will be at or near the maximum the amplifier allows. The range of input voltages in this case will be from less than 1 $\mu$V to 50 $\mu$V or more. If EMGs are to be recorded during movement or isometric tension, then the gain will need to be reduced considerably. EMGs in this application will range upward from 50 $\mu$V to more than a millivolt. Unfortunately, the entire range of activities cannot be usefully recorded at a single gain setting. Small preparatory EMGs are often missed because the attenuation is set so that the largest EMGs occurring during contraction can be recorded without exceeding the limits of the recording system.

As previously stated, the frequency of EMG ranges from about 1 Hz to more than 1,000 Hz, although most of the signal power is between 10 and 150 Hz. If there is a signal-conditioning filter, it should be set for a band pass in this range.

Once the amplifiers are adjusted to the desired gain, a standard calibration signal should be introduced at the input. Some EMG units and polygraphs are equipped with an internal calibration signal. The amplifiers should be adjusted so that calibration signals produce identical output for each amplifier. Calibration signals recorded this way will serve as the basis for quantifying the EMGs.

## Typical Recordings

Figure 8.3 shows the electrode location for recording from the biceps. Figure 8.4 shows the firing of single motor units recorded at high gain from: (a) biceps, (b) lumbricalis, and (c) forehead. In figure 8.5 one can see successive contraction and relaxation recorded from a muscle. Figure 8.6 shows EMG during an arm movement under the following conditions: (a) slow speed, medium-gain, and (b) high speed, high-gain recording of the beginning of movement in (a). Figure 8.6 reveals the differences between high- and medium-gain EMG recording. In Figure 8.6 (a) the EMG can be followed throughout the movement and can be used to document the beginning and end of the movement and something of the effort expended. In figure 8.6 (b) the maximum tension is forfeited in order to be able to examine the developing tension before the movement begins. Figure 8.7 displays frequency histograms of the EMG recorded from the forearm in the following states: (a) relaxation, (b) supporting 100 g, (c) supporting 435 g, (d) during a 30-kg squeeze.

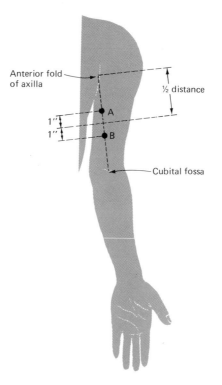

Figure 8.3. Electrode locations for recording from the biceps.

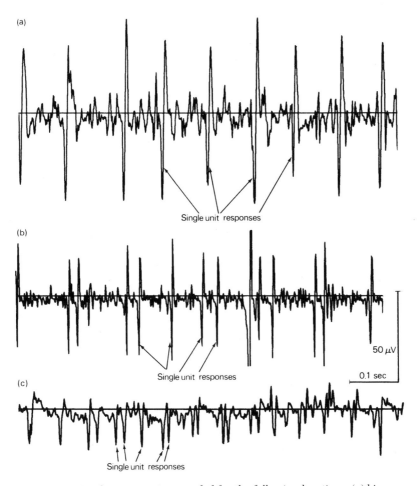

Figure 8.4. Single motor units recorded fro the following locations: (a) biceps; (b) lumbricalis; (c) forehead.

## Common Problems

As is the case with EEG, the appearance of 60-Hz interference in the recorded EMG is by far the most common difficulty. The problem may arise from any of several sources, most of which are discussed in chapter 7. Figure 8.8 displays an EMG from the biceps, the initial part of which is contaminated by 60-Hz noise. In the case of EMGs, the 60-Hz notch filters currently available on many polygraphs should not be used. As may be noted in figure 8.8, 60 Hz is near the center of the most powerful portion of the EMG frequency range, so that eliminating it and attenuating nearby frequencies will distort EMG considerably. Figure 8.9 dem-

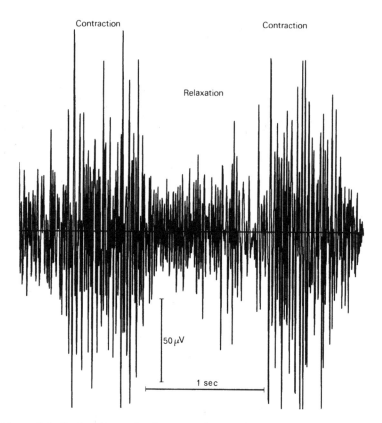

Figure 8.5. Contraction and relaxation of a muscle.

onstrates artifacts generated by movement and by a loose electrode. When interference begins to appear in a previously clear record, the most likely source is a loose electrode or connection.

Other physiologically generated signals may contaminate the EMG. The electrical potential generated by the heart (the EKG) commonly appears, particularly in neck and back leads. This may be overcome by moving the leads closer together or by repositioning the subject. A ground lead attached nearby (not between the two active leads) will often reduce the EKG in the EMG leads. The EKG can often be eliminated by orienting the axis of the EMG electrodes at right angles to the axis of the heart. EEG is clearly present in figure 8.10; the frontal EEG quite reliably contributes to forehead EMG. The EEG is recognizable as a band of low-amplitude, somewhat faster activity. The EEG contribution can be reduced but not eliminated by reducing the space between electrodes to 2 cm or less.

While no obvious distortion appears from incorrect electrode placement, the resulting EMG may not emanate from the intended muscle.

The most common error is to place the two leads of a pair of electrodes at right angles to the fibers of the muscle. This greatly attenuates and distorts the signal, as may be seen in figure 8.11(a), taken from pairs of leads correctly and incorrectly placed over biceps. Alternatively, the two electrodes are sometimes incorrectly placed on different muscles. EMG will then represent the difference between the activity of the two muscle groups rather than that of either one of them. The forehead placement

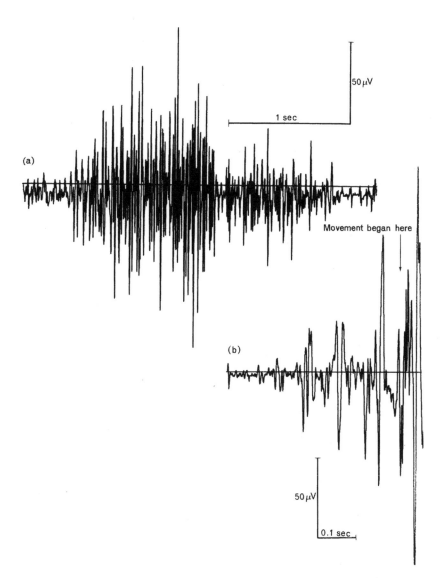

Figure 8.6. EMG during an arm movement: (a) slow speed, medium gain; (b) high speed, high gain.

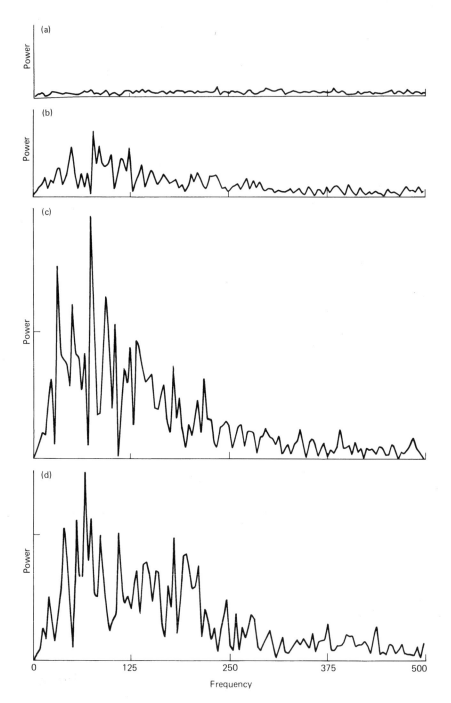

Figure 8.7. Frequency histograms of power in the EMG during four tensions: (a) relaxed arm; (b) 100-g weight; (c) 435-g weight; (d) 30-kg squeeze.

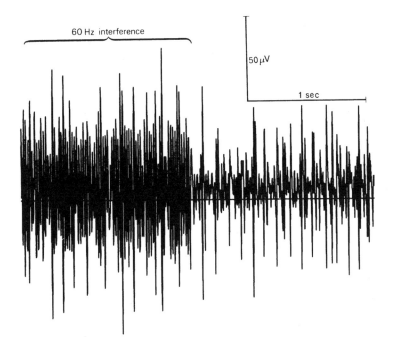

Figure 8.8. EMG recorded from the bicep with 60-Hz interference.

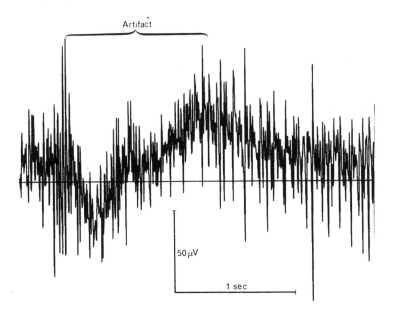

Figure 8.9. Artifacts generated by movement and a loose electrode.

119

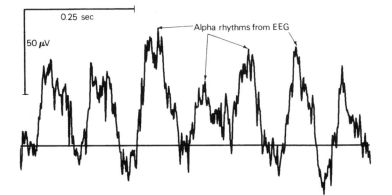

Figure 8.10. EMG recorded from the forehead contaminated with frontal EEG.

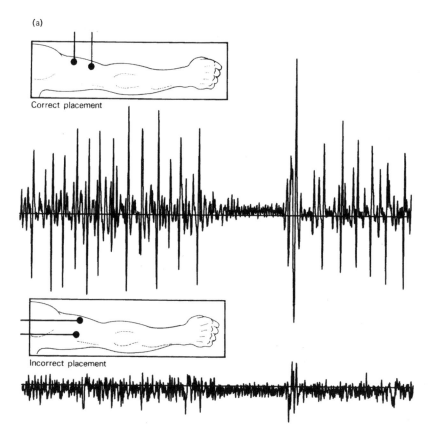

Figure 8.11. EMG recorded with electrodes correctly and incorrectly placed (a) from the bicep;

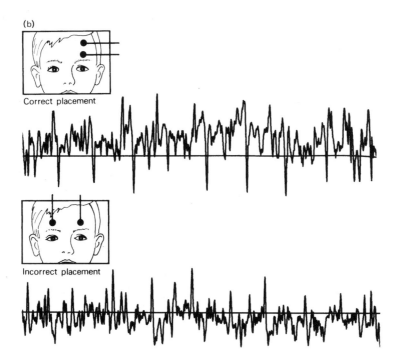

Figure 8.11. (*continued*) EMG recorded with electrodes correctly and incorrectly placed (b) from the frontalis.

suggested by a number of biofeedback practitioners is an example of such a placement and was studied by Davis, Brickett, Stern, and Kimball, 1978. Figure 8.11(b) compares records from these leads to a simultaneously recorded EMG from a single frontalis muscle.

## Analysis and Quantification

In what follows, methods are suggested for the analysis of surface recorded EMGs. Considerable caution must be demonstrated, however, in assigning their muscle origin. It is common to use such terms as "frontalis EMG," or "corrugator" or "buccinator" EMG, for example. But, as indicated earlier, such specific designation is unwarranted because the surface record reflects distant as well as local activity. Particularly in anatomical areas where there are several muscles and where, as is often the case, they are arranged in superficial and deep layers under the same electrode pair, one simply cannot discern which muscle or which combination of them is responsible for the momentary EMG. It is preferable to indicate the position of the electrode in terms of anatomical landmarks.

Nevertheless, EMGs are amenable to quantitative analysis. EMGs, where there is no movement, will usually appear similar to those of figure 8.4. Where discharges of single motor units are recognizable by their amplitude, they may simply be counted, so that an analysis of counts per unit time results. The ultimate limit of this counting procedure occurs when the individual spikes fuse to form the complex waves seen in figure 8.5. Here the analysis of the untreated record becomes very difficult. If

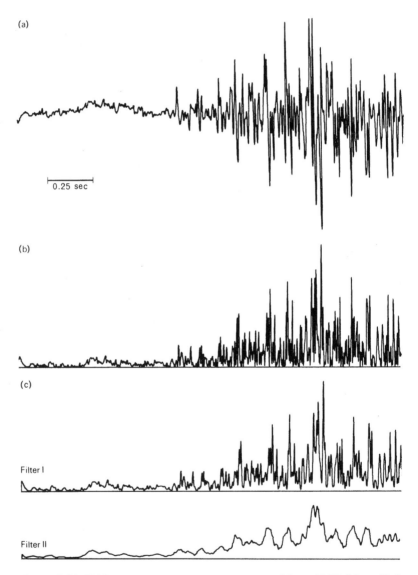

Figure 8.12. EMG preparatory to an arm movement: (a) raw EMG; (b) rectified signal; (c) rectified and filtered using two filters.

the record is divided into equal time segments, various apects of the complex waveform in each may be measured. The largest deflections in each segment, or the average of some number of the largest in each segment, may be used as an approximation of the amplitude of the EMG. These are tedious procedures, and the relation of any single measurement to the tension developed by the muscle is questionable. For these reasons, EMGs are often subjected to considerable alteration within the recorder's output stages.

The most common treatment first specifies the EMG and then integrates the rectified signal. Rectification combines negative and positive deviations around a specified value; it is as though the EMG record was folded lengthwise through the middle of the trace and the underlying waves traced onto the top. Integration of the rectified record with respect to time effectively sums continuously the area above and below the trace, which at any moment represents the absolute EMG amplitude. The integral may be continually displayed or discretely "dumped" onto the polygraph for writeout whenever the integrated voltage reaches some predetermined level. Both integrals permit evaluation of EMGs in terms of amplitude-time relations. As was indicated earlier, the integrated EMG does correspond linearly to muscle tension over a wide range of isometric contractions. Rectification, integration, and filtering can be accomplished by computer as well as in the output stages of the EMG recorder. Figure 8.12 displays: (a) the raw EMG preparatory to arm movement, (b) rectification of the same record, and (c) rectified, filtered EMG using two filters.

Where the EMG is time-locked to an identifiable event, such as an external stimulus or a movement, a researcher can construct averages of many trials of the rectified EMG in a manner identical to that followed for averaged evoked potentials from the brain (see chapter 7).

### References

Basmajian, V. (1963). Control and training of individual motor units. *Science, 141*, 440–441.

Bradley, M. M., Lang, P. J., & Cuthbert, B. N. (1993). Emotion, novelty, and the startle reflex: Habituation in humans. *Behavioral Neuroscience, 107*, 970–980.

Cacioppo, J., Tassinary, L., & Fridlund, A. (1990). The skeletomotor system. In J. Cacopppo & L. Tassinary (Eds.), *Principles of psychophysiology: Physical, social, and inferential elements*. Cambridge: Cambridge University Press.

Darwin, C. (1965). *The expression of emotions in man and animals*. Chicago: University of Chicago Press. (Reprint of edition by D. Appleton & Co, London, 1872).

Davis, C. M., Brickett, P., Stern, R. M., & Kimball, W. H. (1978). Tension in the two frontales: Electrode placement and artifact in the recording of forehead EMG. *Psychophysiology, 15*, 591–593.

Davis, J. F. (1952). *A manual of surface electromyography*. Montreal: Laboratory for Psychological Studies, Allen Memorial Institute of Psychiatry.

Davis, M. (1984). The Mammalian Startle Response. In R. C. Eaton (Ed.), *Neural Mechanisms of Startle Behavior*. New York: Plenum.

Lang, P. J. (1995). The emotion probe. Studies of motivation and attention. *American Psychologist, 50*, 372–385.

Lippold, O. C. J. (1967). Electromyography. In P. H. Venables and I. Martin (Eds.), *A manual of psychophysiological methods*. Amsterdam: North-Holland.

Vrana, S. R., Spence, E. L., & Lang, P. J. (1988). The startle probe response: A new measure of emotion?. *Journal of Abnormal Psychology, 97*, 487–491.

# 9

# Eyes

*Pupillography and Electrooculography*

---

Investigators have claimed that various responses of our eyes can be used to determine a great variety of things, from interest in sexual feelings, to the relative degree of processing occurring in the brain. Some of the more common areas of research have included relating the size of the pupil to arousal and examining eye movements in relation to processes such as reading and dreaming. Of the various measures possible, psychophysiologists have been most interested in *pupillography*, or the measurement of the size of the pupils and eye movement. In this chapter, we will discuss pupillography and *electrooculography*, one technique for studying the position of the eyes.

## Pupillography

In both Eastern and Western cultures, a tradition dating back hundreds of years views the pupils as "windows of the soul." There are stories about merchants who were able to sell their wares by watching the changes in pupil size as the buyer first looked at an item; when the sellers noticed a pupillary response, they knew which item the buyer was really interested in and could set their price accordingly.

Not only has the pupillary response made its way into our folklore, but as Janisse (1977) and Hess (1975) have noted in their brief histories of the area, scientists over the past 200 years have also been intrigued by the response. For example, in the 1870s Darwin related pupillary dilation to emotional responses such as fear and surprise. In the twentieth century there was interest in the pupillary response in different populations, such as children, people with schizophrenia, and groups given various drugs. Although there has been scattered interest in the pupillary response for many years, it was not until the work of Hess in the early

1960s that this response gained the attention of numerous psychologists and other researchers.

Hess (1975) described his first "experiment" in which he showed a series of pictures, including landscapes and a nude female, to his research assistant, James Polt. After a number of pictures, Hess noticed that Polt's pupils became larger in response to the picture of the nude. Following this, Hess and Polt designed other experiments to understand better how psychological stimuli affect pupillary size. The first summary of this research was presented by Hess (1965) in a *Scientific American* article in which he suggested that attraction to a stimulus resulted in pupillary dilation and that pupillary constriction was the outcome of viewing stimuli that were "distasteful or unappealing." Not only did Hess argue that females responded with greater dilation than males to a pleasant stimulus, such as a picture of a mother and baby, but also that people whose pupils were dilated were judged more appealing. He examined this question by showing two pictures of a female to males. The two pictures were identical except that in one picture the pupils were shown to be larger than in the other. Although the males reported that they could not distinguish one picture from the other, they consistently preferred the one with the larger pupils. In the middle ages, the drug belladonna (atropine) was used to produce large-diameter pupils, which were symbolic of beauty in women, hence the name belladonna, "beautiful woman." Janisse (1977) reviewed the work of Hess and others in this area and pointed out that there is still much controversy over the relationship of psychological factors and pupillary responses, especially Hess' aversion-constriction hypothesis.

Although we know that light intensity is a major determinant of the pupillary response, it is the psychological factors including cognitive, emotional, and motor processes that have been of interest to psychophysiologists (see Beatty, 1982; Sirevaag & Stern, 2000, for reviews). For example, when students were asked to commit a mock crime, those with knowledge of the crime scene showed larger pupillary responses to photographs of the scene than individuals without any knowledge of the crime (Lubow & Fein, 1996) In fact, these authors reported that 50% of those who took part in the mock crime and 100% of those who did not could be correctly identified from pupillary responses. Other work suggests that mental effort or mental load also plays a role in pupillary dilation. For example, complex sentences have been shown to produce larger pupillary changes than simple ones (Just & Carpenter, 1993). Likewise, it has been reported that pupil dilation increases as an individual is asked to remember an increasing number of digits (Granholm, Asarnow, Sarkin, & Dykes, 1996). Other intriguing areas of research involving pupillary responses are those involving psychopathology (e.g., Rubin, 1974; Steinhauer & Hakerem, 1992), those examining the interrelationship of pupillary responses with other psychophysiological variables such as heart rate (e.g., Libby, Lacey, and Lacey, 1973; van der Molen, Boomsma, Jennings, & Nieuwboer, 1989), and those that use pupillary responses as a measure of short-term activation during information processing or motor preparation (e.g., Beatty and Wagoner, 1978; Richer & Beatty, 1987). This last area of research has implications for human factors research; that is, pupil diameter can be used to infer work load and fatigue in groups such as airline pilots (cf. Sirevaag & Stern, 1999). For further information, the interested reader should consult the special issue of the *Journal of Psychophysiology, 1991* (3), on pupillary response.

## Physiological Basis

Physiologically, dilation and constriction of the pupil require the involvement of the autonomic nervous system in the following manner. The sympathetic nervous system dilates the pupil through a contraction of the medial fibers of the iris. Parasympathetic activation contracts the circular muscle or the iris and brings about the constriction of the pupil. There are a number of reflexes, as well as other factors, which can bring these responses into play. Tryon (1975) has noted 23 such factors, which are presented in table 9.1. This table points out the complexity of performing carefully controlled studies with this response measure.

## Recording Procedure

*Photographing the Eye*   One of the techniques used by Hess (1972) was photography of the eye with a 16 mm camera. The procedure was as follows. A subject would come into the laboratory, sit down, and look into a boxlike apparatus approximately 2 ft (0.60m) × 2 ft × 2 ft in size. The far side of the apparatus consisted of a screen on which slides could be projected. Mounted on one side of the apparatus was a 16 mm camera aimed at a mirror placed outside of the subject's line of vision which reflected the eye. Hess reported an almost perfect concordance between the pupillary responses of the two eyes and thus suggested that only one eye need be recorded. The pupillary changes were recorded on infrared film, which permitted filming under various lighting conditions and allowed for sharper definition between the pupil and the iris than found with standard negative films. The largest drawback to the filming technique was the film processing time and scoring, usually by hand, which was an expensive and time-consuming procedure. Even a small study required a large number of pupillary measurements. According to Janisse (1977), 20,000 separate measurements would not be unusual; one study used 100,000 measurements. Today, computers allow for easier measurements to be made.

Table 9.1. Sources, and Descriptions, Regarding Variation in Pupil Size

| Sources | Descriptions |
|---|---|
| 1. Light reflex | Pupil constricts with increased intensity of illumination and dilates with decreased intensity of illumination |
| 2. Darkness reflex | Momentary dilation due to interrupting a constant adapting light; different from the light reflex |
| 3. Consensual reflex | Stimulation of one eye affects both eyes equally; failure called dynamic anisocoria. |
| 4. Near reflex | Constriction due to decreasing the point of focus |
| 5. Lid-closure reflex | Momentary contraction followed by redilation |
| 6. Pupillary unrest (hippus) | Continuous changes in pupil diameter |
| 7. Psychosensory reflex | Restoration of diminished reflexes due to external stimulation |
| 8. Age | Decreased diameter and increased variability with age |
| 9. Habituation | Pupil diameter decreases, speed of contraction increases, magnitude of reflex decreases |
| 10. Fatigue | Diameter decreases, amplitude and frequency of hippus increase; age amplifies these effects |
| 11. Alertness and relaxation | Alertness suggestions decrease and relaxation suggestions increase pupil size |
| 12. Binocular summation | Constriction is greater when both eyes are stimulated |
| 13. Wavelength (pupillomotor Purkinje phenomena) | Larger dilation to chromatic than achromatic stimuli; as intensity of illumination is increased, proportionately more constriction is elicited by shorter wavelengths |
| 14. Alcohol | Dilates the pupil in proportion to the percentage of alcohol in the blood |
| 15. Sexual preference | Dilation to sexually stimulating material |
| 16. Psychiatric diagnosis | Abnormal pupillary responses in schizophrenics and neurotics |
| 17. Pupil size | Stimuli involving larger pupils elicit more dilation |
| 18. Political attitude | Dilation for preferred political figures |
| 19. Semantic stimuli | Small pupil diameters associated with high recognition thresholds |
| 20. Taste | Pleasant taste elicits dilation |
| 21. Information processing load | Increasing dilation to increasingly difficult problems |
| 22. Task-relevant response | Having to make a motor response augments pupillary response |
| 23. Incentive | Increases diameter on easy problems only |

*Source:* From W. W. Tryon 1975, "Pupillometry: A survey of sources of variation," *Psychophysiology, 12,* 90–93. Reprinted by permission. Research documenting each factor can be found in Tryon (1975).

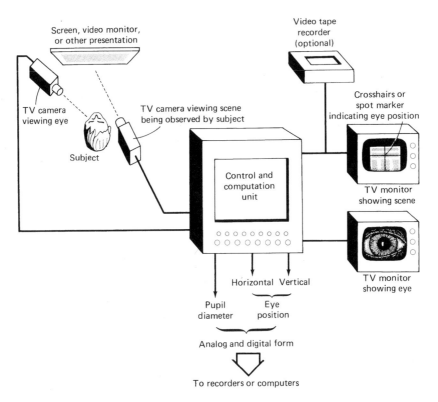

Figure 9.1. Eye monitoring system.

*Electronic Scanning*   Electronic scanning is the most highly developed method for pupillary measurements. One such system is shown in figure 9.1. As can be seen in the figure, the electronic scanning device uses a television camera that records the eye. Most units have a filter that allows infrared light, which cannot be seen by the subject, to be projected on the eye. Within the control unit a special circuit detects the amount of light reflected from the pupil and cornea. The greater the dilation, the less light that is reflected. The television monitor also allows the experimenter to check the picture quality from which the pupil measurement is made for possible artifacts. The television scanning type of system also gives the experimenter immediate feedback concerning the pupillary response.

### Common Problems

Since the measurement of pupillary responses is machine specific, the most common problems, other than gross movements, are related to the manner in which the measurement is taken. Video systems are limited by the scanning rate of the system, which is typically 60 samples per second. There are other problems the researcher should consider, such as whether the system will allow the subject to wear eyeglasses or contact lenses; the maximum amount of head movement the subject can make; how comfortable the subject is; whether the subject can make verbal responses while still giving accurate pupillary data; and so forth. There is one additional problem with television systems which relates to the manner in which the scanner determines the size of the pupil; some systems require extensive calibration for each subject and for a given subject under different conditions.

### Analysis and Quantification

The analysis procedure of Hess (1972) compared the changes in pupillary responses of subjects while they observed a control slide and a stimulus slide, both of which were shown for 10 s. Since both slides were equated for brightness and contrast, Hess interpreted any change in pupillary response to be of an informational or emotional nature. During the control and stimulus situations, about 20 frames of the film were taken for each slide and then analyzed. In his early studies, Hess simply compared pupil area during the showing of the control and stimulus slides. However, in his later work, the measure of percentage change in diameter was used. Television scanning devices use similar measurement units.

## Eye Movements

Eye movement has been used by psychophysiologists to infer cognitive processing. For example, it is possible to record the manner in which good and poor readers move their eyes while reading and to infer from these movements differences in their cognitive approach to the material. Oster and Stern (1980) found that good readers, when changing from general reading to detailed information reading, did not change the length of time between the fixation points but increased the amount of time they paused during each fixation. Poor readers did not change the amount of time they paused; instead, they decreased the amount of material between the fixation points. From the eye-movement records, these researchers were able to infer cognitive processing.

Eye movements have also been used as an indirect measure to infer the presence of dreams, fantasy, and differential processing by the two hemispheres of the human brain. According to the classification system developed by Dement and Kleitman (1957), the initial stages of sleep are characterized by a slowing in EEG frequency and a lack of eye movement. In the so-called fifth stage of sleep, however, a paradoxical phenomenon appears. The person's physiological responses begin to vary more, including an increase in eye movements and a reduction in chin EMG. If someone is awakened during rapid eye movement or REM sleep there is a high probability that dreaming will be reported. In one of the early studies, Dement and Kleitman (1957) reported that 80% of their subjects were dreaming when awakened from REM sleep, whereas only 7% reported dreaming when awakened from non-REM sleep. Thus, for researchers interested in studying subjective factors such as dreaming, fantasy, and flow of consciousness, the measurement of eye movements offers an objective indication of their occurrence.

Eye movement has also been thought to be an indirect measure of hemispheric activation. Based on early work by Day (1964) and Duke (1968), Bakan (1969) suggested that the direction in which one looks after being asked a question is related to the hemisphere of the brain which has been activated in response to the question. The present theory is that right hemispheric activation produces an initial left eye movement, whereas left hemispheric activation produces a right eye movement. This reasoning suggests that by observing eye movement, a researcher can determine which hemisphere is being used in the processing of various types of material. For example, it has been suggested that the left hemisphere is more active in the analysis and production of verbal material, whereas the right hemisphere is more active in the comprehension of spatial and musical material. Research has suggested that there is some validity to this claim, although the total picture is not simple (see Ehrlichman and Weinberger, 1978, for a review of hemispheric activity in relation to eye movements).

Various studies have reported that individuals with schizophrenia display dysfunctions of a particular type of slow eye movement referred to as smooth pursuit (see Clementz & Sweeney, 1990, for a review). The smooth pursuit system allows our eyes to follow relatively slowly moving objects such a pendulum on a clock. Researchers can measure the difference between a target's movement and that of a person's eye movement. In addition to schizophrenics showing pursuit eye movement dysfunctions, studies have reported that first-degree relatives also show dysfunctions. This has suggested to some that eye movement dysfunctions may be a biological marker for schizophrenia.

### Physiological Basis and Classification

*Control of Eye Movement*   Movement of the eye is controlled by six muscles that are innervated by the third, fourth, and sixth cranial nerves. These muscles, working in antagonistic pairs, coordinate movement of both eyes in horizontal, vertical, and circular directions. For example, when both eyes look to the right, the left medial rectus muscles and the right lateral rectus are activated, while the right medial and the left lateral muscles are inhibited. In a similar fashion, vertical movement is controlled by the superior and inferior rectus muscles. The final two muscles, the superior oblique and the inferior oblique, are involved in rotational movements of the eye. Although we have described the three groups of muscles separately, in reality all are involved in each movement of the eye.

*Types of Eye Movement*    As one reads a page of printed material, the eyes move from one fixation point to another. The voluntary jump from one fixation point to another is referred to as *saccadic eye movement*. These movements are fast and characterized by a high initial acceleration and final deceleration. Some scientists have even speculated that the saccade represents the fastest somatic movement that any muscular system in the body can produce.

In contrast to saccades, which are quick, the eyes display slow movements known as smooth pursuit movements. These movements appear not to be under voluntary control and can be elicited by having a person view a moving visual field. Independent of saccadic movements, the smooth movements help to stabilize on the retina the image of the moving object being viewed. In the same manner that smooth movements represent the eye's response to external movement, compensatory movements of the eyes represent movement on the part of the person—either of the head or the body or both.

Another type of eye movement is referred to as *nystagmus movements*, which consist of oscillatory motion of the eye. Specific examples include optokinetic nystagmus, which may be elicited by a moving pattern containing repeated patters; vestibular nystagmus, which may be elicited by head movement that stimulates the semicircular canals; and spontaneous or *gaze nystagmus*, which is an anomaly of the eye related to certain neurological disorders.

Two additional types of eye movements are *torsional eye movements* and *vergence eye movements*. Torsional eye movements are rotational movements about the line of gaze and are smooth and compensatory. Vergence movements are the mechanism by which binocular fixation is maintained. The eyes thus move in opposite directions, so that an object moving toward or away from the eyes always appears as one object. These vergence eye movements are relatively slower than most other types of eye movements. Table 9.2 outlines the various types of eye movements, along with the size, speed, and latency of each.

## Recording Procedure

Eye position, the direction of gaze, and eye movement, or the change in gaze, can be measured by various means. One simple method is to watch the person's eyes or even to record their movement with a movie camera. The problems with just looking include being obstrusive and not obtain-

Table 9.2. Types of Eye Movements

| Type | Description | Size (degrees of arc) | Latency (ms) | Speed (degrees/s) | Possible Recording Methods |
|---|---|---|---|---|---|
| Saccadic movements | Conjugate fast eye movements that carry the eyes from one fixation point to another | 5–50 | 100–500 | 100–500 | Photography<br>Corneal reflection<br>Photoelectric<br>Electrooculography (EOG) |
| Smooth pursuit movements | Conjugate involuntary slow eye movements to follow slowly moving targets | 1–60 | 200 | 1–30 | EOG<br>Photoelectric<br>Photography |
| Compensatory movements | Smooth conjugate involuntary movements used to compensate for passive or active movements of the head or body | 1–30 | 10–100 | 1–30 | Photography<br>Photoelectric<br>EOG |
| Vergence movements | Nonconjugate movements of the eye to maintain binocular vision. Vergence movements are smoother and slower than conjugate pursuit and compensatory movements | 1–15 | — | 6–15 | Corneal Reflection<br>Photography<br>Photoelectric<br>EOG |
| Torsional or rolling eye movements | Involuntary movements around the line of gaze that compensate for the displacement of the visual vertical | — | — | — | EOG<br>Photography<br>Photoelectric |
| Miniature eye movements | Tiny involuntary movements that occur during periods of fixation These methods have been classified into these categories | less than 1 | — | — | Contact lens<br>Corneal reflection |

(continued)

Table 9.2. Continued

| Type | Description | Size (degrees of arc) | Latency (ms) | Speed (degrees/s) | Possible Recording Methods |
|---|---|---|---|---|---|
| Flicks | Sharp saccadic movements | | | | |
| Drifts | Slow movements between flicks | | | | |
| Tremor | Rapid, oscillating movements | | | | EOG |
| Nystagmoid | Eye movements of an oscillating or unstable nature classified into three categories | | | | Photoelectric |
| Ocular or optokinetic | Movement of the eyes in trying to follow a nonhomogeneous field that is continuously moving past the observer | | | | |
| Vestibular | Compensating movements to overcome problems due to impairment of vestibular nerve | | | | |
| Spontaneous or central nystagmus | Occurs when the gaze is directed peripherally and is usually a sign of impairment of the central visual and vestibular pathways | | | | |
| Intraocular movements | Pupillary reflex contraction to change in illumination | | | | Photography |

Source: From B. T. Tursky. 1974. "Recording of human eye movement." In R. F. Thompson and M. M. Paterson (Eds.). Bioelectric recording techniques. New York: Academic Press. Reprinted by permission.
Note: — indicates not applicable.

ing a permanent record of the movements and position for further analysis. A movie camera provides a record of the eyes, but as with pupillary responses, the amount of data to be scored is very large and almost prohibitive. Thus, a number of alternate methods have been developed. We will briefly describe these techniques here; the interested reader should consult Young and Sheena (1975) or Stern and Dunham (1990) for more detailed descriptions.

### Corneal Reflection

One traditional method is the corneal reflection method. The front surface of the cornea acts as a convex mirror to reflect light. Eye position determines the position of the corneal reflection. The reflected light is imaged through a lens onto film, video equipment, or other light-sensitive devices, such as a photo cell. One disadvantage of this device is that it requires the subject's head to remain in a stable position or that head position be calculated for each measurement to ensure an accurate measurement.

### TV Scanning and Other Techniques

Other techniques require scanning of the eye with a television camera. Through the use of photodetectors, the boundary between the iris and the sclera (the limbus) can be detected and the position inferred. Most limbus-boundary techniques, as these are referred to, use infrared light for better illumination of the eye. Another method includes fitting the subject with a contact lens that fits tightly and moves with the eye. Small mirrors are ground into the lens and reflect light onto a recording device. Although contact lenses are one of the most accurate means of eye movement recording, they may impose some discomfort and danger to the subject. Other techniques are also being developed, such as those that use fiber optics. Recently, with the incorporation of online computing systems, video methods of eye movement tracking are becoming more realistic. However, both online video equipment and other techniques with one exception, are beyond the means of most psychophysiological laboratories. The one exception, and the only technique that does not interfere with normal vision, is electrooculography.

## Electrooculography

Electrooculography (EOG) is a method of recording eye movements and position that utilizes equipment commonly found in psychophysiological laboratories. As the name implies, EOG is an electrical technique that records potential differences from electrodes placed around the eyes, the

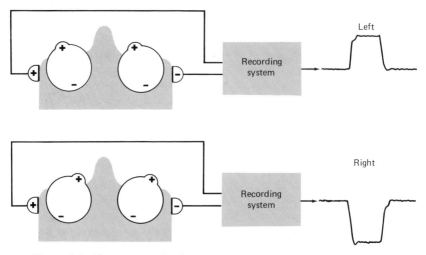

Figure 9.2. The eye as a dipole. Note the movement of the eye and the corresponding tracing on the recording system.

*corneal-retinal potential.* This potential is seen as the result of the difference in potential between the front and the back of the eyeball; that is, the cornea remains 0.40 to 1.0 mV positive with respect to the retina. Thus, the eye may be considered a battery which, as it rotates, carries with it a potential field or dipole which can be measured by placing electrodes on adjacent tissue. This relationship is shown in figure 9.2. This figure shows that, as the eye moves, the potential at the electrode becomes more positive or negative depending upon the direction of movement. EOG can be used to record eye movements up to ± 70°. Typical accuracy is ± 1.5–2.0°.

### Electrodes and Electrode Placement

The most commonly used electrodes for recording eye movements are miniature type (11 mm) silver-silver chloride electrodes; several commercial companies manufacture such electrodes. The electrodes are placed as shown in figure 9.3. Horizontal eye movements are generally recorded with an electrode placed at the outer edge of each eye (outer canthi). It is important to place the electrodes as near to the eye as possible, since the DC potential decreases as the electrodes are placed farther from the eye. Vertical eye movements are recorded with the electrodes above and below the eye. In placing the electrodes, careful alignment is required to eliminate any vertical component in the horizontal measurement, and vice versa. The possibility of cross talk must be further determined by having the subject move the eyes in a horizontal manner and observing the vertical record, and by having the subject move the eyes in a vertical manner and observing the horizontal record. Figure 9.4 shows a record of a subject instructed to move right and left and then up and down. Notice the small amount of cross talk in the two records.

### Procedure

After the subject has been informed about the experimental procedure, the electrodes are placed around the eyes. To insure proper conductance and reduce drift, the skin should be lightly abraded and all excess facial oils removed. Although alcohol is often used when electrodes are placed on other parts of the body, it is suggested alcohol not be used for EOG recordings because of the possible discomfort or damage to the eyes. A cloth or cotton ball wet with water will serve to remove excess oils. Once the electrode site is cleaned, silver–silver chloride electrodes are placed on the skin following standard procedures. That is, when adhesive collars are used, one side is attached to the electrode mount and the electrode cup is filled with electrode paste. Once sufficient paste is applied to insure complete filling, the electrode and collar are attached to the skin, and the leads are connected to the preamplifier and amplifier.

### Recording Equipment

The signal is amplified using a DC amplifier capable of reproducing voltages in the range of 15 to 200 μV. As with any DC amplifier, the use of

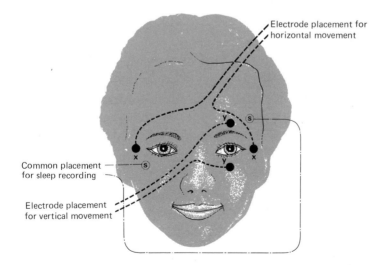

Figure 9.3. Electrode placement for EOG recording of both horizontal and vertical eye movements.

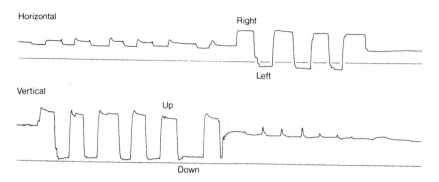

Figure 9.4. Horizontal and vertical eye movement records from a subject who looked first right and then left, and then up and down.

short shielded cable and a high common-mode rejection preamplifier reduces noise. The frequency range of the amplifier depends on the particular eye movement response under consideration. For example, if only eye position is of interest, then it is only necessary to have an amplifier capable of reproducing accurately in the range of 0–15 Hz. If one wishes more exact reproduction of the amplitude of a saccade, then a frequency response of more than 100 Hz is necessary. If one is interested only in the number of saccades, then an AC recording is appropriate, and this eliminates any problem of drift.

### Typical Recordings

Figure 9.5 shows the difference between DC and AC recording of eye movement. Notice that from the DC chart one may derive eye position, but that only the occurrence of a saccade, and not absolute position, can be determined from the AC recording. Figure 9.6 shows horizontal and vertical eye movement recording from a subject who moved the eyes in a circle.

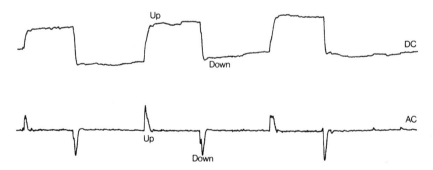

Figure 9.5. DC and AC records of vertical eye movements.

Horizontal

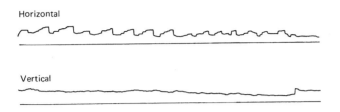

Vertical

Figure 9.6. Eye movement records obtained while an individual's eyes traced a circle.

## Common Problems

There are relatively few problems with the technique just described. The major problem is slow DC drift of the baseline over time. New amplifiers and electrodes make this less of a problem today than previously. Another potential problem, depending upon the nature of the experiment, would be for the subject to change the gaze by turning the head. That is, the subject's eye position would not have changed in relation to the head and thus would not be recorded, but the position would have changed in relation to the environment. This can be prevented by the use of a device such as a chin rest or bite board for keeping the head stable. The chief source of bioelectrical artifacts is muscle potentials. It should also be noted that the potential difference between the retina and the cornea may vary with such factors as light adaptation, diurnal variations, the degree of alertness, and the sex of the subject. These problems are included here to alert the researcher to the complexity of the area and the difficulty of conducting well-controlled studies. For sophisticated applications of eye-movement techniques, the researcher should consult a more detailed reference (Oster & Stern, 1980; Stern & Dunham, 1990; Young & Sheena, 1975).

## Analysis and Quantification

The analysis and quantification of eye movement data vary with the aim of the study. If eye movement is used as a control—as might be the case in an EEG alpha biofeedback study—then one simply looks at the record to determine if the eyes were moving at a particular time. One can likewise look at the record alone to determine saccadic movement and duration during a reading task. If a more precise determination of the orientation of the eyes is required, it is necessary to have performed initial calibrations. That is, the subject should be instructed to look straight ahead, up, down, left, and right at stimuli a known distance away, with each of these points being marked on the EOG record. It is also possible to combine the outputs of the horizontal and vertical traces on a plotter or screen to obtain a representation of where the eyes are looking at any one time. It should be pointed out that the combination of the vertical and horizontal traces may introduce errors that make pinpoint accuracy impossible. These errors may be somewhat reduced by a method of vector EOG recording (Uenoyama, Uenoyama, and Iinuma, 1964). As with any electrophysiological variable, a computer may be used for pattern recognition; the computer then determine the presence, duration, and direction of saccades, or a measure of eye position. Oster and Stern (1980) and Stern and Dunham (1990) describe in some detail the program and hardware used in their studies of eye movement during reading; the interested researcher should consult these reports.

### References

Bakan, P. (1969). Hynotizability, laterality of eye movement, and functional brain asymmetry. *Perceptual and Motor Skills, 28*, 927–932.

Beatty, J. (1982) Task-evoked pupillary responses, processing load, and the structure of processing resources. *Psychological Bulletin, 91*, 276–92.

Beatty, J., & Wagoner, B. L. (1978). Pupillometric signs of the brain activation vary with levels of cognitive processing. *Science, 199*, 1216–1218.

Clementz, B., & Sweeney, J. (1990). Is eye movement dysfunction a biological marker for schizophrenia? A methodological review. *Psychological Bulletin, 108*, 77–92.

Day, M. E. (1964). An eye movement phenomenon relating to attention, thought and anxiety. *Perceptual and Motor Skills, 19*, 443–446.

Dement, W., & Kleitman, N. (1957). Relation of eye movement during sleep to dream activity: Objective method for the study of dreaming. *Journal of Experimental Psychology, 53*, 339–346.

Duke, J. (1968). Lateral eye movement behavior. *Journal of General Psychology, 78*, 189–195.

Ehrlichman, H., & Weinberger, A. (1978). Lateral eye movements and hemispheric asymmetry: A critical view, *Psychological Bulletin, 85*, 1080–1101.

Granholm, E., Asarnow, R., Sarkin, A., & Dykes, K. (1996) Pupillary responses index cognitive resource limitations. *Psychophysiology, 33*, 457–461.

Hess, E. H. (1965). Attitude and pupil size. *Scientific American, 212*, 46–54.

Hess, E. H. (1972). Pupillometrics: A method of studying mental, emotional, and sensory processes. In N. S. Greenfield and R. A. Sternbach (Eds.), *Handbook of psychophysiology*. New York: Holt, Rinehart & Winston.

Hess, E. H. (1975). *The tell-tale eye*. New York: Van Nostrand Reinhold.

Janisse, M. (1977) *Pupillometry: the psychology of the pupillary response*. New York: Hemisphere Publishing Corp.

Janisse, M. P. (1997). *Pupillometry*. Washington, DC: Hemisphere.

Just, M., & Carpenter, P. (1993). The intensity dimension of thought: Pupillometric indices of sentence processing. *Canadian Journal of Experimental Psychology, 47*, 310–339.

Libby, W. L., Lacey, B. C., & Lacey, J. I. (1973). Pupillary and cardiac activity during visual attention. *Psychophysiology, 10*, 270–294.

Lubow, R., & Fein, O. (1982) Pupillary size in response to a visual guilty knowledge test: New technique for the detection of deception. *Journal of Experimental Psychology: Applied. 2*, 164–177.

Oster, P. J., & Stern, J. A. (1980). Electrooculography. In I. Martin and P. H. Venables (Eds.), *Techniques in psychophysiology*. London: Wiley.

Richer, F., & Beatty, J. (1987). Contrasting effects of response uncertainty on the task evoked pupillary response and reaction time. *Psychophysiology, 24*, 258–262.

Rubin, L. S. (1974). The utilization of pupillometry in the differential diagnosis and treatment of psychotic and behavioral disorders. In M. P. Janisse (Ed.), *Pupillary dynamics and behavior*. New York: Plenum.

Shackel, B. (1967). Eye movement recording by electro-oculography. In P. H. Venables and I. Martin (Eds.), *A manual of psychophysiological methods*. Amsterdam: North-Holland.

Sirevaag, E. J., & Stern, J. A. (1999). The gaze control system. In W. Boucsein and R. W. Back (Eds.), *Engineering psychophysiology. Issues and applications*. Mahwah, NJ: Erlbaum.

Steinhauer, S., & Hakerem, G. (1992). The pupillary response in cognitive psychophysiology and schizophrenia. *Annals of the New York Academy of Sciences, 658*, 182–204.

Stern, J. A., & Dunham, N. D. (1990). The ocular system. In J. Cacioppo & L. Tassinary (Eds.), *Principles of psychophysiology: Physical, social, and inferential elements*. New York: Cambridge University Press.

Tryon, W. W. (1975). Pupillometry: A survey of sources of variation. *Psychophysiology, 12*, 90–93.

Tursky, B. T. (1974). Recording of human eye movement. In R. F. Thompson and M. M. Patterson (Eds.), *Bioelectric recording techniques*. New York: Academic Press.

Uenoyama, K., Uenoyama, N., & Iinuma, I. (1964). Vector-electrooculography and its clinical applications. *British Journal of Ophthalmology, 48*, 318–330.

van der Molen, M., Boomsma, D., Jennings, R., & Nieuwboer, R. (1989). Does the heart know what the eyes sees? A cardiac/pupillometric analysis of motor preparation and response execution. *Psychophysiology, 26*, 70–80.

Young, L., & Sheena, D. (1975). Survey of eye movement recording methods. *Behavior Research Methods and Instrumentation, 7*, 397–429.

# 10

## Respiratory System

Respiration refers to the process by which oxygen is supplied to cells and carbon dioxide is removed. The aspects of respiration that psychophysiologists usually measure are breathing rate and amplitude, the latter being a measure of the depth of breathing. The normal rate of respiration in humans is about 12–16 breaths per minute, and the usual depth (*tidal volume*, or total volume of each breath) is about 400–500 ml for healthy adults. Breathing amplitude can be measured either directly (the true volume of the lungs) or indirectly (using a measure such as the circumference of the chest). Some methods of direct volume measurement also allow one to assess the nature and amounts of gases like $CO_2$ that are being expired from the lungs. In addition, one can measure aspects of the respiratory cycle such as the *inspiratory duty cycle* (also called the inspiration fraction) which is the ratio of inspiratory duration to the total respiratory cycle duration. Another measure that provides important information about the influence of the central nervous system on respiration is the *mean inspiratory flow*, which appears to reflect central inspiratory drive and which can be quantified using the ratio of tidal volume to inspiratory duration (Wientjes, 1992).

Relatively few studies in the psychophysiological literature focus on respiration as the response of primary interest, although respiratory manipulations and measures have played a prominent role in studies of anxiety disorders and relaxation (Clark & Hirschman, 1990; Fried, 1993; Papp, Klein, & Gorman, 1993), asthma (e.g., Grossman & Wientjes, 1989; Isenberg, Lehrer, & Hochron, 1992), emotion and stress (Boiten, Frijda, & Wientjes, 1994; Grossman, 1983), and speech (Winkworth, Davis, Ellis, & Adams, 1994). In fact, Wientjes (1992) has suggested that technological advances make respiration measures more useful for psychophysiologists because newer measures provide more information about respiratory function while also being less invasive than older techniques.

When psychophysiologists do record respiration, it is often used as a check for possible artifacts in other response measures caused either by breathing irregularities or by changes in breathing due to an experimental manipulation that might confound (i.e., systematically alter) the measure of interest, such as heart rate. A deep breath, intentional or not, can often bring about a greater change in autonomic nervous system function than will manipulation of the independent variable. For example, Stern and Anschel (1968) had subjects take four different types of breaths and recorded the effects on finger pulse volume, heart rate, and skin resistance. The types of breaths taken are shown in figure 10.1, and the effects on various response measures are shown in figure 10.2. The extent of the ANS disturbance varied directly with the depth of the inspiration, with deeper breaths leading to a decrease in skin resistance, an increase followed by a decrease in heart rate, and vasoconstriction in the finger.

The effect of respiration on heart rate has long been of interest to psychophysiologists. *Respiratory sinus arrhythmia* (RSA) was first described by Ludwig in 1847 (see Daly, 1985), and refers to the rhythmic increases and decreases in heart rate produced by normal respiration in many subjects. As a person inhales, the heart rate increases; as the person exhales, the heart rate decreases (see figure 12.5). Respiratory sinus arrhythmia appears to arise from both afferent connections from the

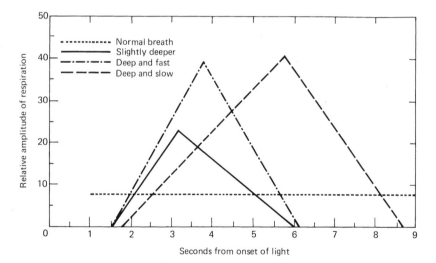

Figure 10.1. Mean relative amplitude of four types of breaths. The graphs are schematic depictions drawn using only the onset, peak, and offset values derived from the original records (which is why they are triangular in shape). For a typical respiratory record, see figure 10.4. Redrawn with permission from R. M. Stern and C. Anschel, 1968, "Deep inspirations as stimuli for responses of the autonomic nervous system," *Psychophysiology*, 5, 132–141.

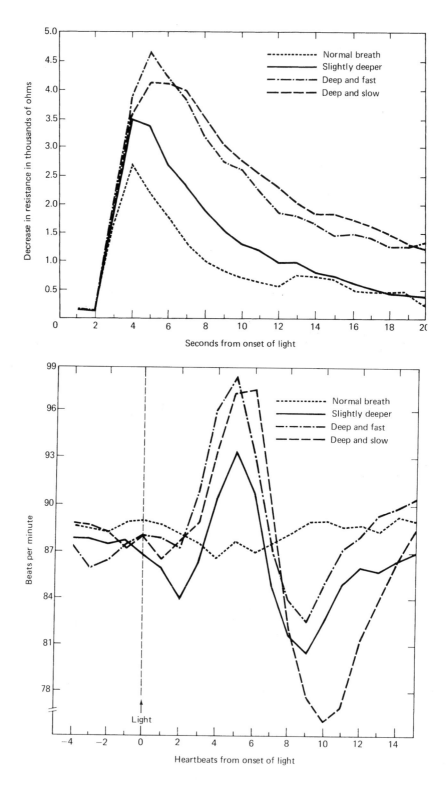

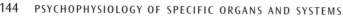

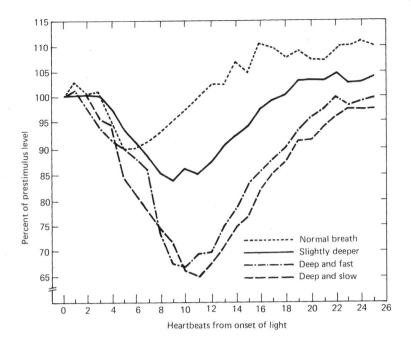

Figure 10.2. Mean group decrease in skin resistance (facing page, top panel), heart rate response (facing page, bottom panel), and finger pulse volume (above) to four respiratory stimuli. Redrawn with permission from R. M. Stern and C. Anschel, 1968, "Deep inspirations as stimuli for responses of the autonomic nervous system," *Psychophysiology*, 5, 132–141.

lungs to the central nervous system (CNS), and from CNS respiratory rhythm generators (Berntson, Cacioppo, & Quigley, 1993; deBurgh Daly, 1985). Respiratory sinus arrhythmia under many circumstances provides a reasonable estimate of the effects of the parasympathetic nervous system on the heart, and is particularly useful to the psychophysiologist because RSA is measured noninvasively. For additional information, see chapter 12.

## Physiological Basis

Respiration is modified by both the central nervous system and the autonomic nervous system, particularly the parasympathetic branch. Respiratory centers in the medulla and pons contain respiratory generator neurons which spontaneously fire bursts of action potentials that initiate inspiration. These brainstem areas have connections to the cortex, the hypothalamus, and other parts of the brainstem. In addition, respiration is also modified by several autonomic reflexes arising from the lungs, upper airways, heart, and blood vessels. For example, if the lungs become overly inflated during inspiration, stretch receptors transmit impulses through the vagus nerve to the brainstem respiratory centers, which then inhibit inspiration and prevent further overinflation of the lungs. This reflex, called the *Hering-Breuer reflex*, does not operate during normal respiration, but appears to protect against overinflation.

Respiratory activity is highly responsive to changes in the concentrations of carbon dioxide and oxygen in the blood. Chemosensitive areas in the brainstem that are part of the respiratory center are directly stimulated by an increase of hydrogen ions in the cerebrospinal fluid, the concentration of which is largely determined by the amount of carbon dioxide in the blood. Although the concentration of oxygen in the blood has no direct effect on the respiratory centers, it is sensed by peripheral chemosensitive areas near the large vessels of the heart. Increases in carbon dioxide sensed by the central chemoreceptors and/or decreases in oxygen sensed by the peripheral chemoreceptors lead to the transmission of impulses to the respiratory center and initiation of inspiration. Interestingly, the level of carbon dioxide is much more important for the regulation of breathing than the level of oxygen. For additional information on the physiological basis of respiration, see Guyton and Hall (1996).

The mechanical changes in the thorax that accompany inspiration and expiration are particularly important for the psychophysiologist because they are noninvasively measurable aspects of breathing. Figure 10.3 illustrates some of the differences in size and shape of the thorax that occur during inspiration and expiration. Just before inspiration be-

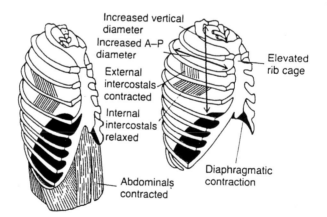

Figure 10.3. Depiction of the ribcage and diaphragm during expiration (left) and inspiration (right). Notice that during inspiration the ribcage is much larger both because the ribs have been lifted up and out and because the diaphragm is more flattened. Redrawn with permission from A. C. Guyton and J. E. Hall, 1996, *Textbook of medical physiology* (9th ed.), Philadelphia: W. B. Saunders.

gins, the diaphragm is relaxed, and in this state, it forms a dome-shaped structure that juts up into the area below the rib cage. Also during this state, some of the muscles (the external intercostals) that attach to adjacent ribs are relaxed, and the ribs will therefore slant downward and forward from their attachments at the spine. When inspiration is initiated, the diaphragm contracts and flattens, which creates a negative pressure in the thorax which forces the lungs open. In addition, the external intercostal muscles contract; this raises the ribs so that they are more nearly perpendicular with the spine, and also pulls the sternum forward. This action causes not only more negative pressure inside the thorax, but also enlarges the circumference of the thorax during inspiration. It is this larger inspiratory circumference that can be measured and used by the psychophysiologist to indicate the phases of respiration. Expiration generally occurs mostly by passive recoil of the chest against the negative pressure created during inspiration. Thus, during expiration, the diaphragm and external intercostal muscles relax, which allows the ribcage to fall down and back toward the spine again. Contraction of the abdominal muscles and activation of the internal intercostal muscles can be used for more active expiration, but these more active processes are not typical for normal, quiet breathing and generally are recruited only during heavy breathing or disease states such as emphysema.

## Recording Procedures

Five methods of recording respiratory variables will be briefly described: *spirometry*, the air-pressure *pneumograph*, impedance pneumography, air temperature, and *respiratory inductive plethysmography*. We will also describe one other method, the strain gauge, in greater detail because it has been (and is likely to continue to be) used often in psychophysiological laboratories.

### Spirometry

A spirometer is a device that measures the volume of air expired with each breath. The subject either breathes through a wide tube, or into a face mask attached to tubing leading to the spirometer. With a nose clip in place to prevent air escaping from the nose, the subject breathes into the spirometer and the volume of air displaced by a breath is measured. Thus, respiratory or tidal volume can be measured directly, and respiratory rate can be derived from the changes in the amount of carbon dioxide that occur over the breathing cycle. Because the nose clip, and face mask or tubing make normal breathing difficult, and also provide resistance to breathing, measurements made with a spirometer are typically considered too intrusive to be used in most psychophysiological studies except for calibration of less invasive measures at one or two time points during an experiment. An example of a study using spirometric measurements is that of Miller and Wood (1994) on air-way reactivity in asthmatic children in response to an emotionally evocative video.

### Impedance Pneumography

Impedance is the opposition to current in an AC circuit and it varies with the volume of a conductor, among other things. The thorax of a breathing subject can be viewed as a conductor when AC current is applied across the chest. The current used to record the impedance pneumograph is very high frequency (typically 20–30 kHz) and cannot harm the subject. The impedance waveforms are produced by the variations in voltage produced by transthoracic impedance changes which occur with each breath. When the lungs are filled with air, impedance of the chest is higher than when the lungs are not full.

As with other indirect respiratory methods, the measure of respiratory amplitude obtained using impedance pneumography is relative and cannot be compared across subjects although indirect methods such as this do yield absolute respiration rate. Using an indirect method, respiratory amplitude is a function of the changes in circumference of the thorax at the specific location where the measuring device is placed. This means that it is not possible to compare amplitude data across subjects or across sessions due to differences in the placement location of the measuring device and body composition of different subjects.

Because the cost of this method is considerably higher than that of the strain gauge method (discussed later) and because the measures of volume obtained are no more accurate than less expensive girth methods, impedance pneumography has not seen wide use in psychophysiology. Recently, suggestions have been made that impedance-derived respiration may be recorded using the impedance cardiograph, which would remove the need for separate electrodes and equipment for measuring respiration if one is already measuring impedance cardiographic waveforms (Ernst, Litvack, Lozano, Cacioppo, and Berntson, 1999; see chapter 12 for more information on impedance cardiography).

### Air Temperature

The air we inhale is cooler than the air we exhale. This difference in temperature is the basis of one method of recording respiration. Either a thermistor or a thermocouple is used to sense changes in air temperature, typically in the vicinity of the subject's nose. *Thermistors* are semiconductors that change resistance with changes in temperature. *Thermocouples* change their voltage output with changes in temperature. Very small thermistors and thermocouples—about the size of the head of a pin—are available, thus making their placement relatively simple. The sensor is typically clipped to the nose or taped in place with the sensor in front of the nostril. The subject breathes in and inhales the relatively cool room air across the sensor; exhaling, the subject warms the air.

Investigators usually report that the subject forgets about the device on or near the nose after a few minutes. This ease of adjustment is important when measuring respiration, since anything that calls the subject's attention to her respiration makes it difficult for her to breathe normally. There is the problem, however, that many subjects breathe partially or even totally through their mouths, making such measures problematic. In addition, any moisture on the temperature-sensitive device (as might happen after a sneeze) will alter the device's sensitivity to temperature. A study, using an air temperature-based device, of the effects of paced respiration on feelings of anxiety was conducted by Clark and Hirschman (1990).

### Respiratory Inductive Plethysmography

A relatively newer measurement of respiratory function developed in the late 1970s has begun to make its way into psychophysiological laboratories. This measure, called respiratory inductive plethysmography, uses AC current to produce changes in self-inductance in coils of wire that encircle the upper chest and abdomen. Self-inductance is the property of a coil of wire that opposes any change in the current that is passing through the coil (it is somewhat analogous to resistance). This property manifests when the voltage applied to a coil changes rapidly, which in turn, produces a change in the current in the coil. Alternations in the direction of current flow (which occur at a frequency of 60 Hz in North America) induce changing magnetic fields around the wires carrying this alternating current. In turn, these changing magnetic fields act to oppose the flow of current in the wire. Self-inductance is partly a function of the cross-sectional area of the coil in which AC current is flowing. For measuring respiration changes, AC current is passed through coils wrapped around the abdomen and thorax, and self-inductance in the coils fluctuates as the cross-sectional area of the thorax changes with each inhalation and exhalation. These respiratory-related self-inductance changes result in variations in voltage output which, when calibrated, are proportional to lung tidal volume.

The measure relies on an assumption that the changes in thoracic cross-sectional area are essentially a function of two components: the volume of the ribcage, and the volume of the abdomen. A ribcage band containing wires in a zig-zag configuration (the coil) is placed over the sternum with the top of the band just below the axillae (the "arm pits"). An abdominal band, also wired in a zig-zag configuration, is placed between the lower ribs and the iliac crests (the anterior protrusions of the hip bones). The voltage output of these two bands together reflects the change in tidal volume, but only after these measures are first calibrated to a spirometer-based volume.

Calibration, generally speaking, is a process whereby a measure without an absolute reference is compared to an absolute reference such that the relative measure can be reported in units of absolute magnitude. In respiratory inductive plethysmography, calibration is performed by simultaneously recording changes in voltage in the abdominal and ribcage coils along with changes in lung volume recorded by a spirometer. Then, as long as the coils do not move during the experiment, the investigator knows how a given change in the voltage output of the abdominal and ribcage bands is related to lung volume. This calibration procedure makes what would otherwise be a relative measure of respiratory amplitude a reasonably good estimate of absolute volume.

Because the equipment is somewhat expensive and requires not only the respiratory inductive plethysmograph but also a spirometer, this technology will likely continue to be used in only a few psychophysiological laboratories. For more information about this technique, the interested reader can refer to Cohn et al. (1982) and Chadha et al. (1982). An example of a psychophysiological study using respiratory inductive plethysmography is found in Winkworth et al. (1994).

### Strain Gauges

One of the most common, and cost-effective, approaches to measuring respiration has been the use of a girth method to measure thoracic circumference (or girth) using a strain gauge. A strain gauge wraps around the thorax and measures the degree of strain placed on the measuring device as the circumference of the thorax increases. As a person inhales, the thorax becomes larger, increasing the stretch on the strain gauge; as the person exhales, the thorax becomes smaller, decreasing the stretch on the gauge. As previously noted for impedance pneumography, girth methods yield only relative measures of respiratory amplitude, and these cannot be compared across subjects unless the amount of stretch is calibrated to a known volume of air displaced by the lungs. Even within a session for a given subject, care must be taken that the strain gauge does not move; if there is any such movement, measures of amplitude recorded early in the session may differ from those recorded later in the same session.

*Transducer.* One commonly used transducer is a length of silastic (synthetic rubber) tubing filled with mercury. The tubing is placed around the chest and a small current is passed through it. As the subject inhales, the cross-sectional area of the mercury in the tube is made smaller, thereby increasing the resistance in the tube. As the subject exhales, the resistance decreases. In a mercury-in-silastic strain gauge, air bubbles can develop in the gauge after several months even if they are not used. Therefore, the continuity, or the presence of an uninterrupted circuit in the gauge should always be checked with an ohmmeter before the gauge is used. Gauges lacking continuity are worthless and must be discarded— and they must be discarded properly because they contain mercury. Fortunately, mercury strain gauges are relatively inexpensive.

Another popular strain gauge device relies on the properties of a piezoelectric crystal material that changes electrical potential when it is deformed. Such crystals are typically placed in a protective plastic device and the crystal is attached to an elastic strap placed around the subject. Deformation of the crystal which occurs when the subject inhales is measured as a change in voltage.

*Transducer Placement.* The respiratory transducer is usually placed around the chest somewhere between the nipple line and the base of the sternum. There is, however, considerable variability as to the point of maximum displacement of the chest or abdomen. It is suggested that the subject take a few deep breaths and the gauge be placed accordingly. Indeed, one problem with recording of respiration only at the abdomen or at the chest is that subjects may change the pattern of breathing within a recording session. For example, someone feeling relaxed may breathe using predominantly abdominal movements, however, if the person became anxious, then she may shift to breathing using primarily chest movements. For these reasons, some investigators prefer to record from two devices simultaneously, one over the chest and one over the abdomen.

*Recording Equipment.* The mercury strain gauge is normally wired into a Wheatstone bridge circuit (see Marshall-Goodell, Tassinary, & Cacioppo, 1990, for details) to obtain a DC voltage output proportional to the resistance change produced by the change in size of the subject's chest with each breath. The specialized respiration couplers that plug into polygraphs are bridge circuits. The signal obtained is relatively large, so a great deal of amplification is not necessary. Piezoelectric devices do not require a bridge circuit, because they produce voltages that can be seen by the polygraph or a computer (although some amplification may be necessary).

*Procedure.* After the subject is seated, the gauge is attached by being stretched slightly and placed around the subject, with the silastic or piezoelectric part in front. For silastic devices, the wires will wrap around the subject's back and they may be held together with an alligator clip behind the subject's back. The gauge can be placed over shirts, blouses, sweaters, and other garments that are not too bulky. The investigator should check to make sure that the belt is tight enough to show deflections with each breath, but not so snug as to be uncomfortable for the subject.

## Typical Recording

A typical recording of respiration is shown in figure 10.4. Inspiration in this illustration drove the pen upward, which is the convention for depicting respiratory traces.

### Potential Problems

A problem that can occur in recording respiration is shown in figure 10.4. When the subject took a very deep breath, the pen went off the recording paper. Obviously, quantification of this portion of the recording would not be possible. These lost data would be no problem if the investigator was interested only in knowing when the subject took a deep breath. However, if one wanted to measure the amplitude of such breaths in the future, one could (a) re-zero the pen so that the point of maximum exhalation on the recording which is almost always the same point, is at the bottom edge of the paper, or (b) reduce the amount of amplification of the signal. In general, respiratory signals collected directly by a computer acquisition program will not have the limitations on range that can be problematic with a polygraph's chart recorder; one must take care however, to make sure that there is sufficient amplification to faithfully reproduce the signal (i.e., so that even shallow breaths can be detected).

Movement of a strain gauge up or down the subject's chest or abdomen will cause what may look like changes in the amplitude of the respiration record and/or a change in the base level (see figure 10.5). In order to minimize such movement, silastic gauges may be taped to the subject's shirt or skin, with one piece of tape placed vertically on each side at the point where the wires pass into the gauge. Care should be taken not to put tape on the gauge itself. For additional information on the use of strain gauges for recording respiratory function, see Lorig & Schwartz (1990).

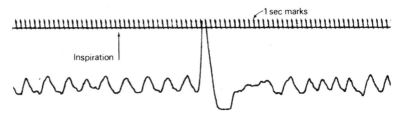

Figure 10.4. Typical recording of respiration with a single deep breath. The upper channel is a timing channel making ticks once per second.

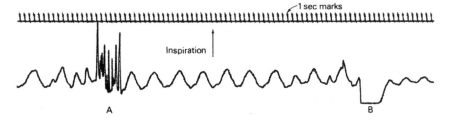

Figure 10.5. Respiratory tracing with timing channel. Point A shows what happens when the subject pulls on or touches the strain gauge. Point B shows a section of the record when the gauge has slipped and loosened.

## Analysis and Quantification

### Respiration Rate

In determining respiration rate, one may score a paper record by hand or use a computer to mark events in the respiratory record and then compute respiration rate. When scoring by hand, the most accurate method is to use a ruler or calipers to measure the distance between several successive cycles (e.g., 30 s or 1 min of data on the polygraph paper) and then divide the number of full cycles within the measured area by the total distance measured. Finally, the researcher converts the measure of the number of cycles/cm into units of breaths/minute using the known chart speed of the polygraph record (e.g., 50 cm/min). This permits the researcher to count how many cycles would occur on average within a 1-min period, even though one did not measure exactly 1 min. With this method, there is no problem of deciding whether or not to include partial cycles at the beginning or end of a measurement epoch.

When scoring respiration using a computer program, it is important to remember that the computer scoring is only as good as the program and the quality of the data input to the program. Typically, respiration rate can be calculated by marking events such as the onset of a breath and the onset of the next breath and converting the duration of a full respiratory cycle into a value of breaths/minute. Alternatively, other places may be marked on the respiratory record, e.g., peaks, which may be better for records where the peaks are more definitive and can be more accurately marked than onsets. Also, it is a good idea to inspect any marks placed by a computer program to see that onsets or peaks are marked accurately. It is not a good idea to assume that the computer is "perfect"; often computer-acquired respiration records are both computer-scored as well as inspected by eye for accurate detection of events in the record.

## Respiration Amplitude

Only the rather invasive technique of spirometry (or calibration of another technique like respiratory inductive plethysmography by spirometry) yields absolute respiratory amplitude values, and these measures are rather uncommon in most psychophysiological studies. For assessing breathing amplitude using relative measures, one can simply measure the amplitude of the inspiratory waveform (using the signal level of the breath at its onset as the baseline) in millimeters and report all experimental comparisons in these arbitrary units. Recall, however, that amplitudes should only be compared within session and within subjects unless calibration to an absolute volume has been performed. As with respiratory rate, amplitude measures can be made by hand or using a computer program. When making amplitude assessments by hand, it is typical to measure the amplitude of a small number of cycles and compute a mean for these chosen cycles. For example, one could take a mean of five pre-stimulus respiratory cycles, and a mean of five poststimulus respiratory cycles and compute a pre-stimulus to poststimulus change in relative respiratory amplitude. When computing respiratory amplitude using a computer, one can typically use the entire record (e.g., compare the entire pre-stimulus period with the entire poststimulus period) because the computer does most of the difficult measurement work.

In addition to measuring amplitude, one can use respiratory amplitude measures to detect very deep breaths or other respiratory irregularities (e.g., a yawn or sneeze) so that subsequent disturbances in ANS response measures can be discounted. One must decide how much deeper than normal the respiration amplitude can be before causing disruptive effects in other measures. As a rule of thumb, it is suggested that if the amplitude of a respiratory cycle is twice as large as or greater than the previous cycle, other psychophysiological responses that occur for at least the next 20 s should be considered "suspect" data.

## Respiratory Events

Respiratory events such as inspiratory time or *inspiratory duty cycle* (the ratio of inspiratory duration to the total breathing cycle) have been used in some studies of respiratory activity. These measures may provide a more complete picture of the workings of the respiratory system. For example, Wientjes (1992) notes that both tidal volume and respiration rate are multiply determined by other features of respiratory function. Thus, respiration rate may increase because of an increase in the inspiratory rate, an increase in expiratory rate, or both. For processes that selectively influence either inspiration or expiration, reporting only the overall respiration rate may lead the investigator to miss a true change in respiratory function. As an example of a process that leads to changes

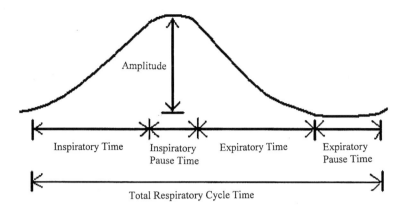

Figure 10.6. Measures of potential interest in a typical respiratory cycle.

in both inspiratory and expiratory times, consider speaking. Speaking can lead to a shortening of inspiratory time because we tend to make a brief, large inhalation just before beginning to speak. In addition, we typically lengthen expiratory time during speech as we exhale air in a slower, more controlled fashion than during normal breathing at rest (Winkworth et al., 1994).

Respiratory events would be scored just as described for respiratory amplitude, with particular points in the waveform marked either by hand or using a computer program. As noted previously, when using a computer to place event markers in the data, it is important to look at the raw data to be sure that there are no abnormalities, and to be sure that marks are being placed at reasonable locations by the computer. Respiratory events that may be of interest to the psychophysiologist are depicted in figure 10.6.

*References*

Berntson, G. G., Cacioppo, J. T., & Quigley, K. S. (1993). Respiratory sinus arrhythmia: Autonomic origins, physiological mechanisms, and psychophysiological implications. *Psychophysiology, 30,* 183–196.

Boiten, F. A., Frijda, N. H., & Wientjes, C. J. E. (1994). Emotions and respiratory patterns: Review and critical analysis. *International Journal of Psychophysiology, 17,* 103–128.

Carry, P. Y., Baconnier, P., Eberhard, A., Cotte, P., & Benchetrit, G. (1997). Evaluation of respiratory inductive plethysmography: Accuracy for analysis of respiratory waveforms. *Chest, 111,* 910–915.

Clark, D. M., & Hirschman, R. (1990). Effects of paced respiration on anxiety reduction in a clinical population. *Biofeedback and Self-Regulation, 15,* 273–284.

Chadha, T. S., Watson, H., Birch, S., Jenouri, G. A., Schneider, A. W., Cohn, M. A., & Sackner, M. A. (1982). Validation of respiratory inductive plethysmography using different calibration procedures. *American Review of Respiratory Diseases, 125,* 644–649.

Cohn, M. A., Rao, A. S. V., Broudy, M., Birch, S., Watson, H., Atkins, N., Davis, B., Stott, F. D., & Sackner, M. A. (1982). The respiratory inductive plethysmograph: A new non-invasive monitor of respiration. *Bulletin Européen de Physiopathologie Respiratoire, 18,* 643–658.

de Burgh Daly, M. (1985). Interactions between respiration and circulation. In N. S. Cherniack and J. G. Widdicombe (Eds.), *Handbook of Physiology: The Respiratory System II* (pp. 529–594). Bethesda, MD: American Physiological Society.

Ernst, J. M., Litvack, D. A., Lozano, D., Cacioppo, J. T., & Berntson, G. G. (1999). Impedance pneumography: Noise as signal in impedance cardiography. *Psychophysiology, 36,* 333–338.

Fried, R. (1993). *The psychology and physiology of breathing.* New York: Plenum.

Grossman, P. (1983). Respiration, stress, and cardiovascular function. *Psychophysiology, 20,* 284–300.

Grossman, P., & Wientjes, C. J. E. (1989). Respiratory disorders: Asthma and hyperventilation syndrome. In G. Turpin. (Ed.), *Handbook of clinical psychophysiology* (pp. 519–554). Chichester: Wiley.

Guyton, A. C., & Hall, J. E. (1996). *Textbook of medical physiology* (9th ed.). Philadelphia: W. B. Saunders.

Isenberg, S. A., Lehrer, P. M., & Hochron, S. (1992). The effects of suggestion and emotional arousal on pulmonary function in asthma: A review and a hypothesis regarding vagal mediation. *Psychosomatic Medicine, 54,* 192–216.

Lorig, T. S., & Schwartz, G. E. (1990). The pulmonary system. In J. T. Cacioppo and L. G. Tassinary (Eds.), *Principles of psychophysiology: Physical, social, and inferential elements* (pp. 580–598). New York: Cambridge University Press.

Marshall-Goodell, B. Tassinary, L. G., & J. T. Cacioppo. (1990). Principles of bioelectrical measurement. In J. T. Cacioppo and L. G. Tassinary (Eds.), *Principles of psychophysiology: Physical, social, and inferential elements* (pp. 113–148). New York: Cambridge University Press.

Miller, B. D., & Wood, B. L. (1994). Psychophysiologic reactivity in asthmatic children: A cholinergically mediated confluence of pathways. *Journal of the American Academy of Child and Adolescent Psychiatry, 33,* 1236–1245.

Papp, L. A., Klein, D. F., & Gorman, J. M. (1993). Carbon dioxide hypersensitivity, hyperventilation, and panic disorder. *American Journal of Psychiatry, 150,* 1149–1157.

Stern, R. M., & Anschel, C. (1968). Deep inspirations as stimuli for responses of the autonomic nervous system. *Psychophysiology, 5,* 132–141.

Wientjes, C. J. E. (1992). Respiration in psychophysiology: Methods and applications. *Biological Psychology, 34,* 179–203.

Winkworth, A. L., Davis, P. J., Ellis, E., & Adams, R. D. (1994). Variability and consistency in speech breathing during reading: Lung volumes, speech intensity, and linguistic factors. *Journal of Speech and Hearing Research, 37,* 535–556.

# 11

## Gastrointestinal Motility

*Electrogastrography*

---

The psychophysiology of the GI system is a relatively unexplored area. This is surprising when one considers the landmark work of Wolf and Wolff (1943) in which they described the secretory and motility changes of their *fistulated* subject to various stress situations, and the recent work of Muth, Koch, Stern, and Thayer (1999) who have demonstrated that behavioral stressors, which influence autonomic and cardiovascular reactivity, also influence gastric activity; there are however, few studies reported in between. But the paucity of psychophysiology research on the GI system is not so surprising when we consider the instrumentation and measurement problems of obtaining data from far inside this constantly changing many-meter-long system.

As a consequence of these problems, no psychophysiological studies of absorption are known to the authors, and few studies of gastric acid secretion have been conducted by psychophysiologists. However, several studies of motor activity have been conducted, particularly in the more easily accessible two ends of the GI tract, the esophagus and rectum, and also in the stomach. In this chapter the major emphasis will be on the motor activity of the stomach as measured with the noninvasive method of electrogastrography.

*Electrogastrography* refers to the recording of electrogastrograms (EGGs). Electrogastrograms reflect gastric myoelectrical activity as it is recorded from the abdominal surface with cutaneous electrodes. EGGs are sinusoidal waves recurring at a rate of 3 cycles per minute (cpm) in healthy humans. This predominant frequency is usually discernable by visual inspection of the signal, but computer analysis is essential for quantitative study of EGG recordings. The stomach is also the source of abnormally fast or slow usually dysrhythmic myoelectrical signals, the *tachygastrias* and *bradygastrias*. Acute or chronic shifts from normal 3 cpm EGG signals to the gastric dysrhythmias are associated with a variety of clinical syndromes and symptoms, particularly nausea. In contrast to the abnormalities in frequency such as the gastric dysrhythmias, the amplitude, duration, waveform, and wave propagation characteristics of the EGG have been infrequently studied.

Psychophysiological and pathophysiological investigations of EGG characteristics in health and disease have increased greatly since the first edition of this book was published. The International EGG Society (IEGGS) was established in 1995, and commercial companies are now selling EGG hardware and software including ambulatory models.

## Physiological Basis

The GI system extends from the mouth to the rectum and includes the mouth, esophagus, stomach, small intestine, large intestine, and rectum. The three functions of the GI system are movement of food through the alimentary tract, secretion of substances that aid in digestion or protect the alimentary tract, and absorption of the digestive end products.

The GI tract may be considered to be a series of muscular tubes that have been modified to perform region-specific digestive functions, that is, transit of food from esophagus to stomach, mixing and emptying of ingested foods from the stomach into the duodenum, and absorption of micronutrients from the small intestine. Other specialized tubes (i.e., the cecum; ascending, transverse, and descending colon; and rectum) conserve water, electrolytes, and nutrients and evacuate wastes. These functions require exquisite control and integration of relevant neural, muscular, and hormonal systems within the GI tract.

The purpose of this section is to describe the relationship of gastric motor activity to gastric myoelectric activity and the EGG. We include more information about the physiological basis of the EGG than we did for the other psychophysiological measures included in this book because we thought that less was known about EGG by most psychophysiologists. Readers desiring additional information about the physiology of the GI system are referred to Johnson, Christensen, Jacobsen, and Schultz (1987), and for more information about EGG the reader is referred to Stern, Koch, and Muth (2000).

### Relationship between Gastric Myoelectric Activity and Gastric Motor Activity

The gastric contractions that occur at 3 cpm during the mixing and emptying of meals are the result of coordinated electromechanical coupling of circular layer smooth muscle cells. What are the electrical and mechanical events within the smooth muscle that underlie the mechanical work performed by the stomach?

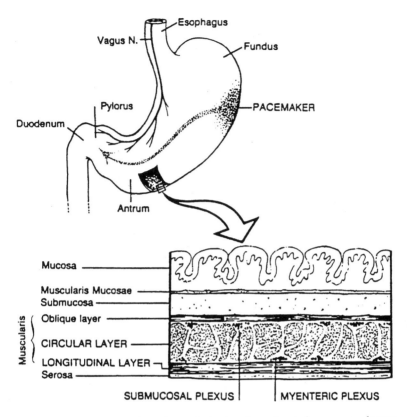

Figure 11.1. The stomach and its principal regions. Inset shows major layers of gastric wall. Origin of gastric pacesetter potentials (pacemaker signals) indicated by stippled region on gastric body. Reprinted with permission from K. L. Koch, 1993, "Stomach." In M. M. Schuster (Ed.), *Atlas of gastrointestinal motility in health and disease*, Baltimore: Williams & Wilkins.

*Gastric Slow Waves*  Gastric slow waves are the electrical events that control gastric contractions. The slow waves result from spontaneous depolarizations of the longitudinal muscle in the region of the juncture of the fundus and body on the greater curvature (see figure 11.1). The outer layer of the circular muscle may participate in the genesis of slow waves. From this region, named the pacemaker area, the depolarization wavefront moves circumferentially and distally toward the distal *antrum*. The normal slow-wave frequency in humans is 3 cpm. The slow wave does not move into the fundic area, which is electrically silent. The slow wave is a spontaneous event, sodium-mediated and omnipresent, and is associated with very low amplitude contractile activity (You & Chey, 1984).

The slow-wave coordinates the frequency and propagation velocity of gastric contractions. That is, the slow wave brings the circular muscle layer near the point of depolarization, and if physical, neural, and/or hormonal signals are appropriate for contraction, the depolarization threshold is reached and circular muscle contraction occurs. Because circular muscle contractions are linked with the slow wave, the circular muscle contractions occur at the slow-wave frequency (3 cpm in humans) and the contractions propagate at the slow-wave velocity (0.8–4 cm/s). For these reasons the slow waves have also been called *pacesetter potentials* and *electrical control activity*. Slow waves are considered myogenic phenomena, but extrinsic neural input may modulate the rhythmicity of depolarization.

*Gastric Spike Potentials*　The electrical events underlying circular smooth muscle contractions are plateau and spike potentials. Depolarization of the circular muscle, in contrast to the longitudinal muscle, is very fast (i.e., spikes). The spikes may or may not occur on plateau potentials, which are associated with the slow wave. The spikes reflect fluxes of calcium passing through the circular muscle membrane. Contractions of the circular muscle may increase tone and/or intraluminal pressure, particularly if they form concentric ring contractions. Such strong contractions may be recorded with strain gauges, intraluminal pressure transducers, or perfused catheters.

In summary, gastric slow waves are present at all times and control the frequency and propagation velocity of spike potentials (i.e., circular muscle contractions) when the latter are elicited by the appropriate stimuli. Gastric slow waves and spike potentials are the myoelectric components of gastric contractions. It is these contractions that perform the work of mixing and emptying foodstuffs. Slow waves and spike potentials from the stomach may be recorded from electrodes sewn to the serosa (the outer surface of the stomach) or from electrodes applied to the gastric mucosa (the inner surface of the stomach). Because slow waves occur within a conducting medium (i.e., the body), they are also recorded with fidelity from electrodes positioned on the skin (i.e., the EGG). Figures 11.2 and 11.3 shows gastric myoelectric activity recorded from serosal and cutaneous electrodes during motor quiescence (figure 11.2) and during gastric peristalsis (figure 11.3).

### Relationship of the EGG to Gastric Myoelectric Activity and Gastric Motor Activity

*EGG and Gastric Myoelectric Activity*　Nelsen and Kohatsu (1968) simultaneously recorded the electrical activity from electrodes implanted on the serosal surface of the stomach and EGGs from 13 patients. They found an excellent correspondence between the frequency of the signals ob-

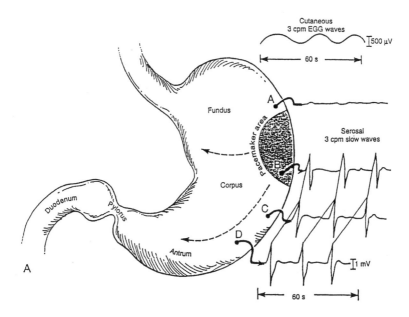

Figure 11.2. Gastric myoelectrical activity during motor quiescence. Pacesetter potentials begin in the pacemaker area located in the proximal gastric body along the greater curve as shown by the darkened area. Slow waves spread circumferentially and distally from the pacemaker region and migrate through the antrum (as shown by serosal electrodes, B, C, and D). The slow-wave migration ends at the pylorus. As the slow wave dissolves in the terminal antrum, another slow wave begins to migrate distally from the pacemaker region. Thus, as shown in the figure, three slow waves will propagate from proximal to distal stomach every 60 s, i.e., 3 cpm slow waves. As shown at point A, the cutaneous electrogastrogram (EGG) reflects the dipole created by the migrating slow wave.

tained from the EGG and the internal electrodes. Another comparison of EGG and serosal recordings from dogs by Smout, van der Schee, and Grashuis (1980b) indicated a perfect correspondence between the frequency of the signals.

In an effort to study the relationship of the EGG to internal electrical activity of the stomach without involving surgery, several investigators have compared the EGG to simultaneously recorded mucosal signals. The mucosal signals are obtained from swallowed electrodes (i.e., electrodes inside the stomach). Hamilton, Bellahsene, Reichelderfer, Webster, and Bass (1986) compared EGG and mucosal signals from 20 human subjects during fasting, after ingesting milk, and in one case, during a period of spontaneous dysrhythmia. They summarized their findings as follows:

> We did find that the surface recordings were of similar visual form as those obtained directly from the mucosa simultaneously. In addition,

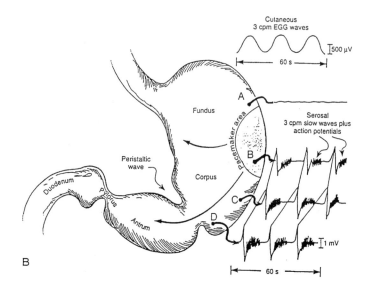

Cutaneous
3 cpm EGG waves

500 μV

60 s

A

Fundus

Serosal
3 cpm slow waves plus
action potentials

Pacemaker area

B

Peristaltic
wave

Corpus

Duodenum

Pylorus

C

Antrum

D

1 mV

B

60 s

Figure 11.3. Gastric myoelectrical activity during gastric peristalsis. Action potentials occur during gastric circular muscle contraction. The action potentials are linked to the gastric slow waves or pacesetter potentials as shown in the extracellular recordings from the serosal electrodes (B, C, and D). As the slow wave linked with action potentials migrates distally along the gastric body and antrum, one gastric peristaltic wave occurs, and one EGG wave is recorded from the surface electrodes. During gastric peristaltic contractions, the EGG amplitude is generally increased. Compare this figure with figure 11.2. Reprinted with permission from K. L. Koch, 1993, "Stomach." In M. M. Schuster (Ed.), *Atlas of gastrointestinal motility in health and disease*, Baltimore: Williams & Wilkins.

frequency analysis determined that the two simultaneously obtained signals were of the same frequency. Finally when the rare arrhythmic events occurred, they were detected in both the mucosal and cutaneous signals. Therefore, the signal obtained from the skin does seem to accurately reflect the BER [basic electrical rhythm] as measured directly from the stomach mucosa (p. 37).

Mintchev, Ott, and Bowes (1997) made simultaneous serosal and EGG recordings from dogs in whom they had created dysrhythmias by surgical means. They reported that the EGG could be used to detect severely abnormal gastric myoelectric activity 93% of the time, and mild abnormalities 74% of the time.

*EGG and Gastric Motor Activity*   Smallwood and his colleagues published a number of studies (e.g., Smallwood, 1978; Smallwood & Brown, 1983) in which they examined the frequency of the EGG and made many advances in techniques for analysis of the EGG signal. In some studies (e.g.,

Brown, Smallwood, Duthie, & Stoddard, 1975) they compared the EGG signal with intragastric pressure recordings. Their findings were the same as those from other laboratories—when contractions occurred, they occurred at the same frequency as the EGG signals; and whereas the EGG showed 3 cpm almost continuously for most subjects, contractions as recorded with intragastric pressure instruments did not.

It should be noted that the simultaneous presence of 3-cpm EGG and the absence of changes in intragastric pressure do not necessarily indicate that the EGG is unrelated to contractions. The possibility exists that the EGG is a more sensitive measure of gastric contractile activity than the pressure-sensitive probes. That is, the EGG may reflect increases in electrical activity (i.e., spike activity) during low-level contractile events that do not alter gastric intraluminal pressure. In fact, Vantrappen, Hostein, Janssens, Vanderweerd, and De Wever (1983) indicated that low-amplitude 5-cpm motor activity is always present in the dog. In addition, You and Chey (1984) have shown that in dogs the 5-cpm pacesetter potentials correlated well with low-amplitude contractions recorded by strain gauges sewn to serosa but correlated poorly with intraluminal pressure changes.

From 1980 to the present, published reports have appeared that not only suggest that the EGG provides information about frequency of contractions but also, indeed, that the amplitude of the EGG is related to the degree of contractile activity (Smout, 1980; Smout, van der Schee, & Grashuis 1980a, 1980b). One of the major contribution of Smout and his colleagues was to point out that the amplitude of the EGG increases when a contraction occurs. They concluded that the pacesetter potential and the second potential, which is related to contractions, are reflected in the EGG. Abell, Tucker, and Malagelada (1985) conducted a study in which they compared the EGG signal from healthy human subjects with the electrical signal recorded from the mucosal surface of the stomach, and intraluminal pressure. They summarized their findings as follows: "Antral phasic pressure activity, when present, was accompanied by an increase in amplitude and/or a change in shape of both the internal and external EGG" (p. 86).

Koch and Stern (1985) reported a close correspondence between the amplitude of EGG waves and the amplitude of peristaltic antral contractions observed during simultaneous EGG-*fluoroscopy* recordings in four healthy subjects. Hamilton et al. (1986) reported that fluoroscopy revealed contractions in the antrum that correlated with three- and four-fold increases in amplitude of the EGG.

The relationship of the amplitude of EGG waves to contractions is complex and not totally understood at this time. However, in addition to the studies mentioned, there is considerable indirect evidence linking amplitude changes in the EGG with strength of contractile activity. For example, in situations where increased contractile activity would be expected (e.g., eating, after swallowing barium), EGG amplitude increases (Hamilton et al., 1986; Jones & Jones, 1985; Koch, Stewart, & Stern, 1987). And in patients with diabetic gastroparesis, where one would expect weak contractility activity, Hamilton et al. (1986) found no increase in the amplitude of EGG after eating.

Can EGG amplitude alone be used to infer reliably the presence or absence of GI contractions? Not at this time. It is possible that with improved methods of measuring contractile activity we will find that all myoelectric activity is accompanied by some contractile activity (see Morgan, Schmalz, & Szurszewski, 1978; Vantrappen et al., 1983; You & Chey, 1984) and that the amplitude of the EGG is related to the intensity or strength of contractile activity. A significant question then becomes: Can the amplitude of the EGG be used to determine whether the accompanying gastric contractile activity is of sufficient strength to do the motor work of the stomach, i.e., mixing and propelling?

Several investigators (e.g., Bruley, des Varannes, Mizrahi, Curran, Kandasamy & Dubois, 1991; Dubois and Mizrahi, 1994) have been examining the possibility of using the EGG as an indirect measure of gastric emptying. Chiloiro, Riezzo, Guerra, Reddy, and Giorgio (1994) simultaneously recorded gastric emptying using ultrasound and the power in the normal 3-cpm EGG from healthy subjects. The correlations ranged from 0.68 to 0.96. Other investigators (e.g., Chen, Richards & McCallum, 1993) have demonstrated a negative relationship between the presence of dysrhythmias in the EGG and gastric emptying. And Bortolotti, Sarti, Barara, and Brunelli (1990) have demonstrated the presence of tachygastria in patients suffering from idiopathic gastroparesis, that is, patients with severely delayed gastric emptying with no known cause.

In summary, the frequency of the EGG is identical to the frequency of gastric pacesetter potentials recorded from the mucosal or serosal surface of the stomach. There is no general agreement, however, on the interpretation of the amplitude of the EGG. Indirect evidence from several studies has demonstrated that amplitude increases during an increase in contractile activity; however, the amplitude of the EGG alone cannot be used to determine the presence or absence of contractions.


## Recording Procedure

### Electrodes

Silver-silver chloride electrodes should be used. The size is not important, but the electrical stability is. Since a relatively small, very slowly varying potential will be recorded, the electrodes should show little bias or, as some refer to it, offset potential.

## Electrode Placement

EGG recording is done with bipolar electrodes placed on the skin surface usually over the antrum of the stomach, plus a reference electrode on the right side of the subject's abdomen. The optimal recording sites will depend on the nature of the signal desired: e.g., largest possible amplitude; lowest artifact from EKG, respiration and subject movement; and the position of the subject's internal organs, particularly the antrum of the stomach and the diaphragm (Mirizzi & Scafoglieri, 1983). The exact placement of the electrodes is not important if the frequency of the EGG is what is of interest, and it usually is. In fact, the EGG can be recorded from the subject's two wrists, but the amplitude will be low compared to recordings from the abdomen because the wrist electrodes are far from the source of the signal, namely, the gastric pacemaker in the antrum. For good EGG recordings from most subjects we recommend placing one active electrode on the subject's left side approximately 6 cm from the midline and just below the lowest rib. The second active electrode should be placed on the midline just above the umbilicus. The reference electrode may be placed anywhere on the right side of the subject's abdomen.

## Recording Equipment

The EGG is a relatively weak and slow biological signal. Therefore, a high-quality recording system is needed that can amplify and process a 100–800 μV signal in the frequency range of 0.5–15.0 cpm. Polygraphs with the appropriate amplifiers can record the EGG. In addition, several companies make appropriate amplifiers and analog-to-digital boards that prepare the EGG signal for analysis, with the proper software, on a PC. Ambulatory EGG equipment is also available that stores the data on a memory card for later analysis. Whatever equipment is used, it is important to have a visual display of the raw signal so that you can be confident that a good signal is being processed.

## Procedure

Subjects should be instructed what and when to eat prior to an EGG recording session because the contents of the stomach will effect the EGG. For most studies, we instruct subjects to fast for at least four hours prior to the experimental session. In other studies subjects are asked to come to the lab after an overnight fast and are given a standard small breakfast such as two pieces of toast and juice. The best EGG recordings will be obtained if the subject lies supine (that is, on the back) or reclines in a comfortable chair. If the subject must move, ambulatory recording equipment should be used with Fetrodes, which are miniature preamplifiers that are attached to the electrodes and reduce movement artifacts. If more than one recording system is available, EGGs may be taken simultaneously from multiple abdominal locations using a single reference electrode. Prior to the attachment of the electrodes, the subject's skin must be prepared by shaving away hair (if excessive), abrading, and cleaning with alcohol.

## Typical Recordings

### Eating and Sham Feeding

A number of investigators have reported that eating a nutritive meal increases the amplitude or power of normal 3-cpm activity and produces a brief frequency decrease. Figure 11.4 shows a typical EGG recording from a healthy subject prior to and after eating. Note the increase in the amplitude and regularity of the normal 3-cpm signal after eating.

Stern, Crawford, Stewart, Vasey, and Koch (1989) have used a *sham feeding* procedure to examine cephalic-vagal influences on the EGG. Following a 15-min baseline period, subjects were required to chew and expectorate a hotdog and roll. After another 10-min baseline period, subjects were given a second hotdog to eat normally. The effect on the EGG of eating the hotdog was as expected: a large increase in the amplitude of the 3-cpm EGG wave that lasted several minutes. The effect on the EGG of sham feeding was an equally large but short-lasting

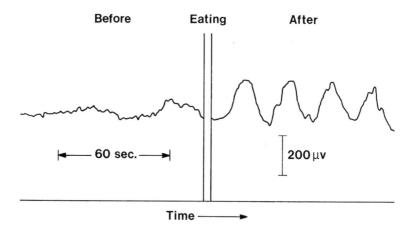

Figure 11.4. Effects of eating on the EGG. Note the increase in amplitude and regularity of the 3 cpm activity after eating.

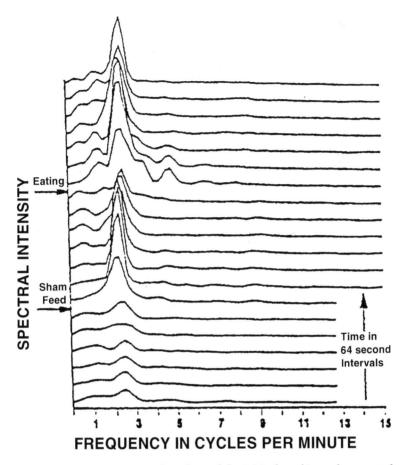

Figure 11.5. Running spectral analysis of the EGG of a subject who reported that the experience of sham feeding was not disgusting. Note the low level of activity at approximately 2.5 cpm before sham feeding and the increase in power during sham feeding and during eating.

increase in the amplitude of the EGG. The EGG of a typical subject from this study is depicted in figure 11.5 as a running *spectral analysis.* The use of such analyses will be discussed in the section on Analysis and Quantification: for now, however, note that frequency is plotted on the X axis, time on the Y axis, and power is the third dimension that seems to rise from the page. This type of plot is referred to as a pseudo-three-dimensional (3-D) plot. It was of interest to note that two subjects who reported after the session that the experience of chewing and expectorating the hotdog was disgusting showed a decrease rather than an increase in the amplitude of their EGG during sham feeding (see figure 11.6).

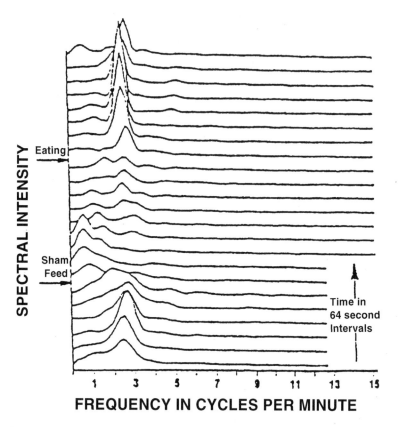

SPECTRAL INTENSITY

Eating

Sham
Feed

Time in
64 second
Intervals

FREQUENCY IN CYCLES PER MINUTE

Figure 11.6. Running spectral analysis of the EGG from a subject who reported that the experience of sham feeding was disgusting. This subject showed power at approximately 2.8 cpm before sham feeding and a decrease during sham feed. The subject showed the typical increase in power during eating. Reprinted with permission from R. M. Stern, H. E. Crawford, W. R. Stewart, M. W. Vasey, & K. L. Koch, 1989, "Sham feeding. Cephalic-vagal influences on gastric myoelectric activity," *Digestive Diseases and Sciences, 34,* 521–527.

## Cold Pressor Test

Stern, Vasey, Hu, and Koch (1991) examined the effects of the cold pressor test on EGG activity. A subject who had recently eaten was asked to put one hand into a container of ice water (4°C) for 1 min, take it out for 15 s, put it back for 1 min, and so on, for a total of 20 min. Figure 11.7 shows the running spectral analysis of the EGG from a typical subject from this study. As can be seen, there was a significant attenuation of EGG 3-cpm activity starting at the point in time when the subject put one hand in ice water. Tachygastria was not seen in response to the cold pressor test, a procedure that induces pain in addition to stress.

## Motion Sickness

In the first experiment that attempted to relate changes in gastric myo-electric activity to the development of symptoms of motion sickness, Stern et al. (1985) obtained EGGs from 21 healthy human subjects who were seated within an optokinetic drum, the rotation of which produced vection (illusory self-motion). Fourteen subjects developed symptoms of motion sickness during rotation, and in each subject the EGG frequency shifted from the normal 3 cpm to 4–9 cpm, indicating tachygastria. Figure 11.8 shows an example of the EGG recording of one of these subjects. Note that the frequency of the subject's EGG was 3 cpm prior to drum rotation, but it changed to 6 cpm (tachygastria) after about 4 min of rotation. The subject reported nausea after 6 min and requested that the drum be stopped after 11 min. In six of seven asymptomatic subjects, the 3-cpm EGG pattern was unchanged during rotation. Figure 11.9 shows a portion of one of these EGG recordings. It was concluded from this and several subsequent studies that the sensory mismatch created by the illusory self-motion produced tachygastria and symptoms of motion sickness in susceptible subjects.

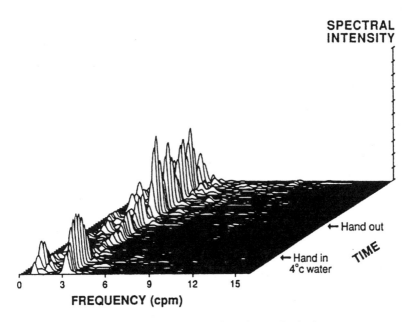

Figure 11.7. Running spectral analysis of a subject who had eaten just prior to putting one hand in ice water. Note the inhibition of 3 cpm power when the subject put the hand in the cold water and the gradual recovery. Reprinted with permission from R. M. Stern, M. W. Vasey, S. Hu, & K. L. Koch, 1991, "Effects of cold stress on gastric myoelectric activity," *Journal of Gastrointestinal Activity, 3,* 225–228.

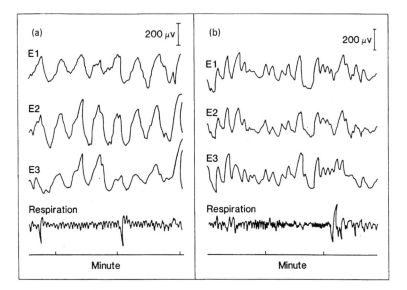

Figure 11.8. (a) EGG activity recorded from upper, middle, and lower electrodes (E1–E3) prior to drum rotation. The EGG frequency is 3 cpm. (b) EGG from same subject after start of drum rotation. Note presence of tachygastria (6 cpm). Tachygastria began at 4 min, and the subject reported nausea at 6 min. At 11 min, he requested that drum rotation be stopped. Reprinted with permission from R. M. Stern, K. L. Koch, H. W. Leibowitz, I. Lindblad, C. Shupert, & W. R. Stewart, 1985, "Tachygastria and motion sickness," *Aviation, Space and Environmental Medicine, 56,* 1074–1077.

## Common Problems

A quick deflection usually indicates that the subject moved, disturbing the subject-electrode interface. A slow drift in one direction for a minute or more usually indicates electrode or amplifier malfunction.

The most obvious thing to check if an EGG recording is flat or almost flat is to see if there is sufficient amplification and a proper band-pass filter. Keep in mind that you are recording microvolts not millivolts, and if the subject has considerable fat between the stomach and the electrode, the normally weak signal will be further attenuated. Also be aware that if the subject has not eaten for several hours, the readings might show very low amplitude EGG because the stomach is quiescent.

In some cases a strong respiratory signal will dominate the EGG. It is not possible to filter out the respiratory signal because its frequency is too close to that of the EGG. The extent to which respiration is seen in an EGG record depends on how close the diaphragm of the subject is to the stomach. This will vary from subject to subject and will also depend on the subject's posture. The basic problem is that in some cases the subject's stomach moves with each breath, producing the unwanted respiratory artifact in the EGG. The only sure way to know if an EGG signal with a frequency at 10–15 cpm is being generated by the stomach or intestines or by respiration is to record respiration separately.

## Analysis and Quantification

### Spectral Analysis

Spectral analysis is currently the most commonly used method of quantifying the EGG signal. Spectral analysis typically uses the Fast Fourier Transform (FFT) to convert a signal in the time domain into the frequency domain using a series of coefficients describing the amplitudes and phase relationships of its independent sinusoidal waveforms. This transformation is analogous to a prism transforming white light into the visible spectrum of colors. (See chapter 14 for more about FFT and signal analysis.)

The output of a spectral analysis is the squared magnitude of the Fourier transform and is typically graphed as a curve showing the

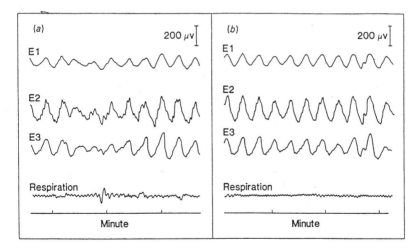

Figure 11.9. (a) EGG activity prior to drum rotation. The EGG frequency is 3 cpm. (b) The EGG from the same subject 7 min after start of drum rotation. Subject reported no symptoms of motion sickness and the EGG frequency remained 3 cpm during 15 min of drum rotation. Reprinted with permission from R. M. Stern, K. L. Koch, H. W. Leibowitz, I. Lindblad, C. Shupert, & W. R. Stewart, 1985, "Tachygastria and motion sickness," *Aviation, Space and Environmental Medicine, 56,* 1074–1077.

strength, or power, of the frequencies into which the original signal can be decomposed. Although power has a very specific meaning in mathematics and physics, we may think of it as an index of the amplitude of the sine waves of a particular frequency that would be required in order to recreate the EGG record. In the analysis of EGG recordings we are usually interested in the power within the following three frequency bands: 0–2.25, 2.5–3.5, and 3.75–9.75. The exact cutoffs for these bands vary from lab to lab. The first frequency band represents the often found but poorly understood ultra slow rhythm referred to as bradygastria. The second encompasses the normal electrical rhythm of the healthy human gastric antrum (3 cpm). The third includes frequencies commonly associated with nausea and is referred to as tachygastria when regular, and gastric tachyarrhythmia when dysrhythmic.

Van der Schee, Smout, and Grashuis (1982) have described an extension of this method that uses running spectral analysis to depict EGG data. Running spectral analysis, with overlapping power spectra displayed as a function of time, yields both frequency and time information. The more conventional spectral analysis provides power only as a function of frequency, not time. With running spectral analysis, frequency, power, and time can be depicted two-dimensionally either with a pseudo 3-D display or with a grayscale plot. Figures 11.5 and 11.6 show two examples of running spectral analyses, and Figure 11.7 shows an additional example.

A brief description of the procedure used to convert raw EGG data to a pseudo-3-D display follows. The first step in any quantification procedure is to insure that quality data are being analyzed. Hence, time must be taken to insure the quality of EGG recordings before complex analysis procedures are undertaken. For single-channel recording for most subjects see our recommendation in the section on Electrode Placement. The amplifying and recording system should filter out signals below 0.5 cpm and above 15 cpm. With these filter settings one can record ultra slow rhythms (0.5–2.0 cpm) but still eliminate shifts in baseline due to DC potentials. Frequencies higher than 30 cpm are filtered out to avoid domination of the gastric signal by EKG. Respiration can also obscure the EGG but its frequency range falls near that of tachygastria and, rather than remove it with analog filters at the time of the recording, it is preferable to remove it later with more precise and flexible digital filters or by using a separate respiration recording to select visually and exclude data that contain respiration artifact.

From the amplifier the EGG signal goes to an analog-to-digital (A/D) converter where it is digitized into a series of numerical values representing discrete voltage levels of the input signal. Thus the analog EGG signal is converted to a digital time series that can then be subjected to a wide range of analyses. A/D conversion units typically allow sampling at a wide range of speeds. Given an EGG signal which has had frequencies faster than 15 cpm or .25 Hz attenuated at the time of recording, a sampling rate of at least 1 Hz is required. We recommend a sampling rate of 4.267 Hz, which yields 256 data points per minute.

Once the EGG signal has been digitized, it must be preprocessed in order to meet the assumptions of spectral analysis. Because the dominant frequency in the EGG is relatively slow, we recommend the use of at least 4-min data windows. Thus, at 4.267 samples per second, a 4-min segment would be composed of 1,024 data points. It is generally desirable to center data for spectral analysis around a mean of zero. This is easily accomplished by subtracting the mean of the segment from each data point. Additionally, the EGG is likely to contain some very slow components that reflect a shifting baseline or other undetermined factors. Such extremely low frequency shifts and simple linear trends should be removed to provide a clean spectrum. A high-pass digital filter which attenuates frequencies below .01 Hz will accomplish such trend removal. One can also remove simple linear trends by fitting a least-squares regression line and subtracting it from the data segment.

After preprocessing, the data segment is Fourier transformed and the spectral density estimates calculated. In order to produce a running spectral analysis, one should overlap consecutive data segments by, for example, 75%. In other words, segment 1 includes minutes 1–4, segment 2 includes minutes 2–5, etc. Thus, 1 min of new information is provided in each consecutive power spectrum. These overlapping power spectra can be plotted in a pseudo-3-D fashion to allow easy viewing of changes in power at various frequencies as a function of time (see figures 11.5, 11.6, and 11.7).

While such running spectral analyses do provide a useful way to view frequency and power changes over time, it is important to note that transient changes in the EGG may go unnoticed if they are small. If such transient changes are large enough they will appear but only as a gradual change with the peak in spectral density appearing in the pseudo-3-D display several minutes after it occurred in real time. Thus, running spectral analysis may not be appropriate for experiments in which very short duration stimulus induced changes are expected. For such cases adaptive spectral analysis methods are recommended; see, for example, Lin and Chen (1994). Similarly, spectral analysis is useful only when the EGG signal contains a significant amount of cyclical activity. This is usually the case for 3-cpm activity, but some gastric phenomena occur intermittently and may not appear in a spectral plot. For more appropriate methods of analysis for quantification of very brief duration, intermittent phenomena, see, for example, Hölzl, Loffler, and Muller's (1985) discussion of so-called zoom FFTs, and Lin and Chen's (1994) discussion of the exponential distribution.

Once spectral power estimates have been calculated, data reduction is usually performed. Our lab typically calculates percentage of total power estimates for the bradygastria, normal 3 cpm, and the tachygastria bands previously mentioned. This is accomplished by summing the power estimates for a given band, dividing this sum by the total spectral power, and multiplying by 100%. However, when looking at changes in percentage of power as a function of, for example, exposure to a stressor, the calculations of percentage of 3-cpm activity and tachygastria can be grossly distorted if there is a large change in the amount of bradygastria. In such cases we recommend calculating the ratio of power in the normal 3-cpm and tachygastria bands before and after presentation of the stimulus. Various other methods of data reduction can be found in the literature. Chen and McCallum (1991) have proposed focusing on the frequency peak which contains the dominant power of the EGG signal. It is possible to analyze both changes in the power of this peak and changes in the frequency of the dominant peak. Smout, Jebbink, and Samson (1994) have suggested an instability factor, which is essentially a measure of the frequency variability of this dominant peak. The best method for reducing the EGG frequency and power data from an FFT is still unsettled. In most cases it will depend on the question to be answered and all of the previously mentioned methods have merit.

## Future Directions

EGG, because of its noninvasive nature, will continue to aid basic researchers in their quest for additional information about gastric myoelectric activity, gastric motility, and their relationship in normal and pathophysiological conditions. Applied research using the EGG by gastroenterologists is increasing rapidly largely due to the ease and reliability of its use in detecting gastric dysrhythmias and the recently established relationship between gastric dysrhythmias and upper GI disorders including delayed gastric emptying and nausea. Much of this research has been supported by pharmaceutical companies, and we anticipate that this will continue. A related exciting new area that requires EGG recording in order to assess results is electrical pacing of the stomach. Research is currently being carried out on dogs and on a small number of humans in cases of gastric paresis where the stomach has ceased contracting and no drugs are helpful. A less dramatic but related area of research that we have planned is biofeedback of EGG for individuals with gastric dysrhythmias in an effort to restore normal 3-cpm activity and thereby relieve nausea. The recent increase in the use of the EGG by gastroenterologists has brought with it refinements in both hardware and software, including ambulatory units that have flown on space shuttle flights. We predict that with the availability of this new equipment additional psychophysiologists will soon be using the EGG to study the effects of stress and emotions on gastric activity.

## References

Abell, T. L., Tucker, R., & Malagelada, J. R. (1985). Simultaneous gastric electro-manometry in man. In R. M. Stern & K. L. Koch (Eds.), *Electrogastrography: Methodology, validation, and application* (pp. 78–88). New York: Praeger.

Bortolotti, M., Sarti, P., Barara, L., & Brunelli, F. (1990). Gastric myoelectrical activity in patients with chronic idiopathic gastroparesis. *Journal of Gastrointestinal Motility, 2,* 104–108.

Brown, B. H., Smallwood, R. H., Duthie, H. L., & Stoddard, C. J. (1975). Intestinal smooth muscle electrical potentials recorded from surface electrodes. *Medical and Biological Engineering, 13,* 97–103.

Bruley des Varannes, S., Mizrahi, M., Curran, P., Kandasamy, A., & Dubois, A. (1991). Relation between postprandial gastric emptying and cutaneous electrogastrogram in primates. *American Journal of Physiology, 261,* 248–225.

Chen, J., & McCallum, R. W. (1991). Electrogastrogram: Measurement, analysis, and prospective applications. *Medical and Biological Engineering and Computing, 29,* 339–350.

Chen, J., Richards, R., & McCallum, R. W. (1993). Frequency components of the electrogastrogram their correlations with gastrointestinal motility. *Medical and Biological Engineering and Computing, 31,* 60–67.

Chiloiro, M., Riezzo, G., Guerra, V., Reddy, S. N., & Giorgio, I. (1994). The cutaneous electrogastrogram reflects postprandial gastric emptying in humans. In J. Z. Chen & R. W. McCallum (Eds.) *Electrogastrography: Principles and applications* (pp. 293–306). New York: Raven Press.

Dubois, A., & Mizrahi, M. (1994). Electrogastrography, gastric emptying, and gastric motility. In J. Z. Chen & R. W. McCallum (Eds.), *Electrogastrography: Principles and applications* (pp. 247–256). New York: Raven Press.

Hamilton, J. W., Bellahsene, B. E., Reichelderfer, M., Webster, J. H., & Bass, P. (1986). Human electrogastrograms. Comparison of surface and mucosal recordings. *Digestive Diseases and Sciences, 31,* 33–39.

Hölzl, R., Loffler, K., & Muller, G. M. (1985). On conjoint gastrography or what the surface gastrograms show. In R. M. Stern & K. L. Koch (Eds.), *Electrogastrography: Methodology, validation, and applications* (pp. 89–115). New York: Praeger.

Johnson, L. R., Christensen, J., Jacobsen, E. D., & Schultz, S. G. (Eds.). (1987). *Physiology of the gastrointestinal tract.* New York: Raven Press.

Jones, K. R., & Jones, G. E. (1985). Pre- and postprandial EGG variation. In R. M. Stern & K. L. Koch (Eds.), *Electrogastrography: Methodology, validation, and applications* (pp. 168–181). New York: Praeger.

Koch, K. L. (1993). Stomach. In M. M. Schuster (Ed.), *Atlas of gastrointestinal motility in health and disease.* Baltimore: Williams & Wilkins.

Koch, K. L., & Stern, R. M. (1985). The relationship between the cutaneously recorded electrogastrogram and antral contractions in man. In R. M. Stern & K. L. Koch (Eds.), *Electrogastrography: Methodology, validation, and applications* (pp. 116–131). New York: Praeger.

Koch, K. L., Stewart, W. R., & Stern, R. M. (1987). Effects of barium meals on gastric electromechanical activity in man: A fluoroscopic-electrogastrophic study. *Digestive Diseases and Sciences, 32,* 1217–1222.

Lin, Z., & Chen, J. Z. (1994). Comparison of three running spectral analysis methods. In J. Z. Chen & R. W. McCallum (Eds.), *Electrogastrography: Principles and applications* (pp. 75–98). New York: Raven Press.

Mintchev, M. P., Otto, S. J., & Bowes, K. L. (1997). Electrogastrography can recognize gastric electrical uncoupling in dogs. *Gastroenterology, 112,* 2006–2011.

Mirizzi, N., & Scafoglieri, V. (1983). Optimal direction of the electrogastrographic signal in man. *Medical and Biological Engineering and Computing, 21,* 385–389.

Morgan, K. G., Schmalz, P. F., & Szurszewski, J. H. (1978). The inhibitory effects of vasoactive intestinal polypeptide on the mechanical and electrical activity of canine antral smooth muscle. *Journal of Physiology, 282,* 437–450.

Muth, E. R., Koch, K. L., Stern, R. M., & Thayer, J. F. (1999). Effect of autonomic nervous system manipulations on gastric myoelectrical activity and emotional responses in healthy human subjects. *Psychosomatic Medicine, 61,* 297–303.

Nelsen, T. S., & Kohatsu, S. (1968). Clinical electrogastrography and its relationship to gastric surgery. *American Journal of Surgery, 116,* 215–222.

Smallwood, R. H. (1978). Analysis of gastric electrical signals from surface electrodes using phase-lock techniques. Part 2: System performance with gastric signals. *Medical and Biological Engineering and Computing, 16,* 513–518.

Smallwood, R. H., & Brown, B. H. (1983). Non-invasive assessment of gastric activity. In P. Rolfe (Ed.), *Non-invasive physiological measurements.* Vol. II. London: Academic Press.

Smout, A. J. P. M. (1980). *Myoelectric activity of the stomach: Gastroelectromyography and electrogastrography.* Thesis, Erasmus University, Rotterdam.

Smout, A. J. P. M., van der Schee, E. J., & Grashuis, J. L. (1980b). Postprandial and interdigestive gastric electrical activity in the dog recorded by means of cutaneous electrodes. In J. Christensen (Ed.), *Gastrointestinal motility* (pp. 187–194). New York: Raven.

Smout, A. J. P. M., Jebbink, H. J. A., & Shannon, M. (1994). Acquisition and analysis of electrogastrographic data: The Dutch experience. In J. Z. Chen & R. W. McCallum (Eds.) *Electrogastrography: Principles and applications* (pp. 3–30). New York: Raven Press.

Smout, A. J. P. M., van der Schee, E. J., & Grashuis, J. L. (1980a). What is measured in electrogastrography? *Digestive Diseases and Sciences, 25,* 179–187.

Stern, R. M., Koch, K. L., Leibowitz, H. W., Lindblad, I., Shupert, C., & Stewart, W. R. (1985). Tachygastria and motion sickness. *Aviation Space, and Environmental Medicine, 56,* 1074–1077.

Stern, R. M., Crawford, H. E., Stewart, W. R., Vasey, M. W., & Koch, K. L. (1989). Sham feeding: Cephalic-vagal influences on gastric myoelectric activity. *Digestive Diseases and Sciences, 34,* 521–527.

Stern, R. M., Koch, K. L., & Muth, E. R. (2000). Gastrointestinal system. In J. T. Cacioppo, L. G. Tassinary, & G. G. Berntson (Eds.), *Handbook of Psychophysiology* (pp. 294–314). Cambridge: Cambridge University Press.

Stern, R. M., Vasey, M. W., Hu, S., & Koch, K. L. (1991). Effects of cold stress on gastric myoelectic activity. *Journal of Gastrointestinal Motility, 3,* 225–228.

van der Schee, E. J., Smout, A. J. P. M., & Grashuis, J. L. (1982). Applications of running spectrum analysis to electrogastrographic signals recorded from dog and man. In M. Wienbeck (Ed.), *Motility of the digestive tract* (pp. 241–250). New York: Raven.

Vantrappen, G., Hostein, J., Janssens, J., Vanderweerd, M., & De Wever, I. (1983). Do slow waves induce mechanical activity? *Gastroenterology, 84,* 1341.

Wolf, S., & Wolff, H. G. (1943). *Human gastric function.* New York: Oxford University Press.

You, C. H., & Chey, W. Y. (1984). Study of electromechanical activity of the stomach in humans and in dogs with particular attention to tachygastria. *Gastroenterology, 86,* 1460–1468.

# 12

# Cardiovascular System

*Heart Rate; Cardiac Output; and Blood Pressure, Volume, and Flow*

The heart is a muscle, referred to as the myocardium, which begins functioning within the fourth week of embryonic development and continues to beat 3 billion to 4 billion times throughout life. About the size of a fist, the heart weighs less than a pound and contracts about 60–75 times a minute. As it beats, the heart moves blood to various organs, including the lungs (pulmonary circulation), the heart (coronary circulation), and the rest of the body (systemic circulation). Psychophysiologists have long been interested in the functioning of the heart and circulation and have focused their attention on such measures as heart rate, blood pressure, blood volume, and blood flow. This chapter will discuss the recording and analysis of these and related measures, after providing a brief overview of cardiovascular physiology.

## Physiological Basis

The heart consists of a left and right pump, each with two chambers, the atrium and the ventricle. The right pump supplies blood to the pulmonary system, and the left pump supplies oxygenated blood to the rest of the body. Venous blood, low in oxygen, returns to the heart and enters the right atrium. Contraction of the right atrium forces blood into the right ventricle. The right ventricle then contracts, forcing blood into the lungs through the pulmonary artery. Blood oxygenated in the lungs enters the left side of the heart. The blood is pumped from the left atrium into the left ventricle. From there, the contraction, or systolic action of the heart muscle, forces the blood into the aorta, the major artery of the heart, for distribution throughout the body. Distribution of blood throughout the body is accomplished by a system of arteries, smaller vessels referred to as arterioles, and capillaries. Blood returns to the heart through the veins. At rest, the majority of the blood is in the veins, which act as reservoirs.

The amount of blood pumped by the heart per unit time is referred to as *cardiac output*. At rest, the cardiac output is approximately 5 liters per minute, but this amount may increase 400% to 600% during extreme exercise. There also is a change in the distribution of blood during exercise. For example, at rest, the muscles receive only 15% of the cardiac output, with the brain receiving 14%, and the kidney and liver receiving 22% and 27%, respectively. However, with extreme exercise, muscles may receive 75% of the total blood flow. This shift of blood flow during exercise is controlled in part by the sympathetic nervous system (SNS). Thus, sympathetic innervation causes vasoconstriction in some parts of the body, which provides more blood for use at the muscles. In addition, local metabolic effects of lowered oxygen at the muscles leads to vasodilation in the vessels of the exercising muscles. These vasodilatory effects appear to occur because of the release of humoral (fluid-borne) substances that are presumably released from the tissues that need additional oxygen. In summary, humoral factors are released in response to the local nutritional needs of the tissues of the body, whereas SNS innervation directs the overall distribution of blood.

The SNS shifts blood flow not only during exercise but also in response to temperature changes of the body, postural changes, and strong emotional responses such as fear. For example, if body temperature becomes elevated, inhibition of the SNS produces a vasodilation of the arterioles of the skin. This in turn increases the flow of warm blood to the skin, with a resulting heat loss. When a person changes posture, blood is also shunted to particular areas of the body to maintain blood pressure. When a person stands from a seated position, a drop in blood pressure is registered at pressure sensors called *baroreceptors* in the chest and neck. These sensors send a message to the brainstem, which activates the SNS throughout the body and results in vasoconstriction in the peripheral blood vessels which returns the blood pressure to prestanding levels. Fear and other strong emotions can also result in increased sympathetically mediated vasoconstriction, and this activation is specific to particular vascular beds. For example, Anderson, Wallin, and Mark (1987) showed that during a mental arithmetic task, activity increased in muscle sympathetic nerves innervating the leg, but did not increase muscle sympathetic outflow to the arm. Thus, sympathetic activity makes an important contribution to the redistribution of blood flow when the body's needs change, and this redistribution is directed very precisely to reduce blood flow to certain vascular regions and provide additional blood flow to areas with the greatest need. It should be pointed out that the parasympathetic nervous system (PNS) is generally considered to have a relatively minor effect on the blood vessels.

Vasoconstriction and vasodilation change the resistance to blood flow through the vessels. This change in resistance directly affects both blood flow and blood pressure. This relationship, the physiological analog to Ohm's law, states that blood flow through a vein or artery equals the difference in pressure between the two ends of the vessel divided by the resistance to the flow of blood. Thus, the resistance of a constricted vessel would be greater than that of a dilated one and a vessel with high resistance will have slower blood flow and higher pressure than a vessel with low resistance. This relationship holds not only for individual vessels but also for the entire body, and may be written as follows:

Cardiac Output (amount of blood pumped per unit of time) = Arterial Blood Pressure / Total Peripheral Resistance (resistance of all vessels in the systemic circulation).

## Electrical Activity of the Heart

The electrical activity of the heart as recorded at the surface of the skin is measured by a technique known as *electrocardiography*. The printed record is called the electrocardiogram or EKG. (The abbreviation EKG is derived from the German spelling, but the abbreviation ECG is sometimes also used.) A typical EKG is illustrated in figure 12.1. A careful reading of an EKG can discern how electrical activity spreads across the muscle of the heart. The *sinoatrial node* (S-A node) is a small strip of muscle located in the upper part of the right atrium. It is at this point that the initial impulse begins that triggers the contraction of the heart. The cells of the S-A node are also referred to as pacemaker cells because of their ability to originate an electrical impulse. The electrical impulse passes from the S-A node through the atria to the *atrioventricular node* (A-V node). With this passage, the atrial muscle depolarizes; this is represented in the EKG by the P wave. Mechanical contraction of the atria follows depolarization after a brief (ms) interval. At this point, the blood is being passed into the ventricles. The impulse is delayed briefly (about 0.09 s) in the A-V node, allowing time for the atrial contraction to produce complete ventricular filling. It then passes through the common bundle of His and into the ramifications of the Purkinje network. These fibers transmit the impulse almost immediately through the ventricular system and result in blood being pushed into the lungs and body. It is the depolarization of the ventricles that produces the characteristic QRS complex so predominant in the ECG. The ventricles then repolarize; this is represented by the T wave of the ECG. The precise relationships between each component of the ECG are a valuable aid in determining disorders of the heart, such as premature ventricular contractions, sinus bradycardia, fibrillation, and tachycardia. Some abnormal rhythms, or arrhythmias, are

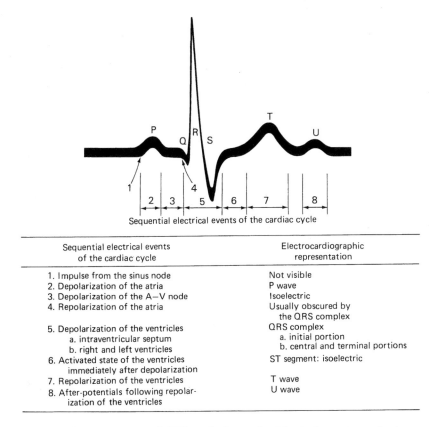

Sequential electrical events of the cardiac cycle

| Sequential electrical events of the cardiac cycle | Electrocardiographic representation |
|---|---|
| 1. Impulse from the sinus node | Not visible |
| 2. Depolarization of the atria | P wave |
| 3. Depolarization of the A–V node | Isoelectric |
| 4. Repolarization of the atria | Usually obscured by the QRS complex |
| 5. Depolarization of the ventricles<br>    a. intraventricular septum<br>    b. right and left ventricles | QRS complex<br>    a. initial portion<br>    b. central and terminal portions |
| 6. Activated state of the ventricles immediately after depolarization | ST segment: isoelectric |
| 7. Repolarization of the ventricles | T wave |
| 8. After-potentials following repolar- ization of the ventricles | U wave |

Figure 12.1. Prototypical EKG and electrophysiological events producing characteristic features of the EKG. Redrawn with permission from R. Philips and M. Feeney, 1973, *Cardiac rhythms*, Philadelphia: Saunders.

shown in figure 12.2. High heart rate (tachycardia) or low heart rate (bradycardia) may be a function of numerous conditions, which include pathology as well as factors related to diet, posture, exercise, emotional excitement, and mental activity. The last two factors have been of particular interest to psychophysiologists.

## Cardiac Responding

Early studies on the effects of stressors on the cardiovascular system suggested that there was a strong and concerted action of the sympathetic nervous system in response to potent stressors such as fear stimuli. This systemwide increase in sympathetic activational effects on the cardiovascular system produced concurrent increases in heart rate and blood pressure as well as other "arousal-related" responses such as increased ac-

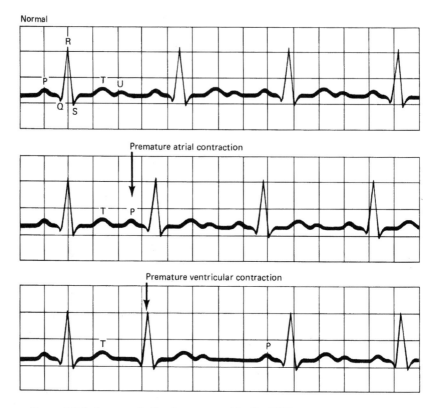

Figure 12.2. Some arrhythmias apparent in the EKG.

tivity of the sweat glands (i.e., increased skin conductance) and increased breathing rate. However, research with more mild to moderate stressors has demonstrated much greater variety in the patterns of cardiovascular responding, suggesting that the concept of a unitary "arousal" response pattern is misleading. Beatrice and John Lacey and their colleagues showed that so-called arousal responses in visceral organs controlled by the autonomic nervous system did not always occur in concert with one another, and were determined in large part by the situation or context in which these responses occurred (Lacey, 1967; Lacey, Kagan, Lacey, & Moss, 1963). The Laceys noted that on some occasions changes in the heart rate and skin conductance were inversely related, so that heart rate decreases were accompanied by skin conductance increases. Such a pattern of differential responsiveness in two or more physiological systems being controlled by the autonomic nervous system was referred to as *directional fractionation* and has been observed extensively across physiological systems. For a further discussion of these issues, see chapter 5. Also as an offshoot of their work on visceral responses to sensory stimuli and environmental stressors, the Laceys derived an intake-rejection hypothesis of cardiac responding which suggested that cardiac deceleration permits sensory information to be processed more effectively, whereas cardiac acceleration promotes the rejection of or inattention to intense, unpleasant, or painful sensory stimuli. This hypothesis is somewhat counterintuitive because it proposes that a peripheral physiological system can affect the central nervous system, rather than the other way around. Later work by Obrist and colleagues questioned the role of heart rate in producing an attentive state because pharmacological blockade of the cardiac deceleration preceding a reaction time response did not prevent the participant from producing a quick response (Obrist, Webb, Sutterer, & Howard, 1970). These data, however, do not preclude the possibility that changes in blood pressure, rather than heart rate, may provide feedback to the central nervous system and either facilitate or inhibit sensory processing. Indeed, neurophysiological evidence supports the idea that blood pressure increases can blunt the perception of pain, as well as inhibit sensorimotor activity and reflex action. The mere presence of feedback signals from the periphery to the central nervous system does not necessarily mean that the feedback to the central nervous system is sufficiently potent under normal physiological conditions to provide any useful information to the organism. Thus, we do not yet know whether heart rate deceleration or blood pressure decreases are simply outputs of an "attentive" nervous system or whether they may be causally related to altered attentional abilities.

Changes in the cardiovascular system are also linked to motor activity, and bodily movement is typically accompanied by an increase in heart rate. This phenomenon is known as *cardiac-somatic coupling* (Obrist, 1981, 1982). Movement demands blood flow to fulfill the metabolic needs of skeletal muscle activity. This does not imply, however, that cardiac changes occur only in response to changes in metabolic need, and indeed, cardiac changes in excess of metabolic requirements occur frequently, a phenomenon called additional heart rate (Turner, 1994). Preparatory cardiac responses, especially to novel situational demands, appear to be common and may represent an attempt by the body to be ready for whatever challenge is forthcoming. After repeated presentations of a situational demand, the cardiac response is typically titrated more closely to the actual metabolic needs of the demand; that is additional heart rates are smaller with succeeding presentations of a demand.

One can see from figure 12.3 that the heart is innervated by both the sympathetic and parasympathetic branches of the ANS. Activation of the parasympathetic nervous system results in a decrease in heart rate, whereas a decrease in parasympathetic activity results in an increase in heart rate. Conversely, an increase in sympathetic activation of the heart results in an increase in heart rate and the force of contraction of the heart (contractility), whereas a decrease in sympathetic activation to the heart decreases heart rate and contractility. Although the two branches

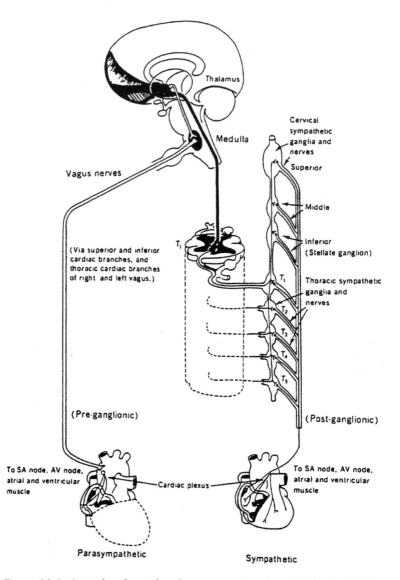

Figure 12.3. Central and peripheral nervous system input to the heart. This figure illustrates both the parasympathetic (left side) and sympathetic (right side) autonomic inputs to the heart. (Reprinted by permission from J. F. Green, 1987, *Fundamental cardiovascular and pulmonary physiology*, 2nd ed., Philadelphia: Lea & Fibiger,

often act in a reciprocal fashion to control the heart such that activity in one autonomic branch increases while activity in the other autonomic branch decreases, this reciprocal relationship between the two branches does not invariably characterize cardiac control (Berntson, Cacioppo, & Quigley, 1991). Under some circumstances, activity in both autonomic branches may increase (or decrease) concurrently (a coactivational mode); in other cases, activity in one branch may change while activity in the other branch does not (an uncoupled mode). See chapter 5 for further discussion of this issue. Because basal heart rate as well as changes in heart rate may arise from different combinations of autonomic nervous system activity, heart rate alone can not reveal the underlying activity of the ANS. For this reason, cardiovascular researchers interested in understanding the contributions of the ANS to heart rate activity must combine measures of autonomic effects on the heart with those of heart rate.

## Measures of Autonomic Effects on the Heart

*Respiratory Sinus Arrhythmia*   Respiratory sinus arrhythmia (RSA) is an oscillation in heart period due to the respiratory cycle (Porges, 1986; Berntson et al., 1997). Changes in RSA appear to reflect the activity of the vagus nerve, and an increase in RSA is strongly positively correlated with increases in parasympathetic influence on the heart. RSA is measured by assessing how much heart period changes from beat to beat. One simple way it can be measured is by using the maximal difference (in ms) between the heart period associated with inspiration and the heart period associated with expiration (peak-valley method). During inspiration, heart period is shorter than during expiration and this difference in heart period across the respiratory cycle can index parasympathetic changes. Fast Fourier Transform (FFT) or other methods (e.g., the Porges and Bohrer method; Porges & Bohrer, 1990) can also assess the degree of oscillation in heart period from beat to beat that falls within the respiratory frequency. These techniques can provide similar results to those using the peak-valley method (Grossman, van Beek, & Wientjes, 1990). For additional information on the physiological basis and measurement of RSA, see Berntson et al. (1997) and Berntson, Cacioppo, & Quigley (1993). For additional information on techniques such as FFT, see chapter 14.

*Pre-ejection Period*   One of the most promising estimates of sympathetic effects on the heart currently seems to be the systolic time interval known as the *pre-ejection period* (PEP). This is the time between the electrical signal to the ventricles initiating contraction and the ejection of blood from the left ventricle into the aorta. PEP can serve as an estimate of sympathetic influences on the heart because it usually reflects changes in cardiac contractility (or the force of contraction). PEP is negatively correlated with sympathetic activity. One must use caution, however, in making inferences about PEP because it also may change with large hemodynamic alterations such as when a person changes posture (in this case, the change in PEP is not related only to sympathetic influences on the heart). PEP is measured using two devices simultaneously, the EKG and impedance cardiography. The impedance cardiograph permits a researcher to record when changes in the velocity of blood flow occur in the thorax—in particular, those associated with the ejection of blood flow into the aorta. For further information on the measurement and sympathetic basis of PEP see Berntson et al. (1994), Newlin and Levenson (1979), and Sherwood, et al. (1990).

## Heart Rate or Heart Period

### Recording Procedure

Although the electrical activity of the heart had been noted previously, it was not until the start of the twentieth century that a device capable of faithfully reproducing this activity was developed. This instrument was developed in Holland by Willem Einthoven, who is the founder of modern electrocardiography. Einthoven's device, the string galvanometer, continued in use until the advent of vacuum tube amplifiers in the 1930s and 1940s. Einthoven also experimented with other aspects of EKG work, including various types of electrodes. He was later awarded the Nobel Prize for this work.

*Electrodes and Their Placement*    The first electrodes used for EKG recording were buckets of saline solution in which the arms and legs were immersed. Silver-silver chloride electrodes are commonly used today. Although there exists a standardized system for electrode placement on the limbs and chest utilized for medical diagnosis, all that is required for an EKG of sufficient quality to measure heart rate is that two electrodes be placed on the skin fairly far apart. Psychophysiologists use standard limb leads designated as follows: I, one electrode on each arm; II, right arm and left leg; III, left arm and left leg (see figure 12.4). An electrode placement which is less sensitive to body movement than standard limb leads entails placing electrodes on the torso with one electrode on the distal end of the right collarbone and the other on the lower left rib cage. This has been referred to as a modified Lead II placement because the resulting EKG is very similar to that obtained by a Lead II recording made from the limbs (figure 12.4). This placement minimizes artifacts due to move-

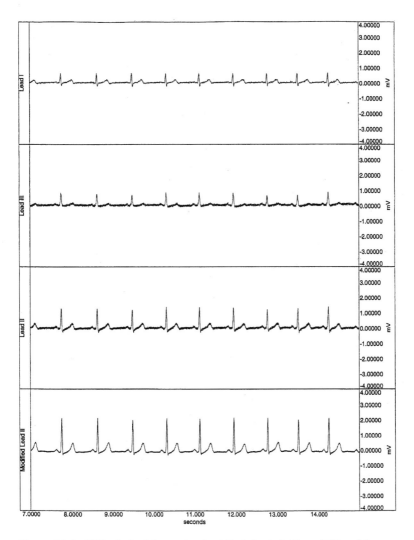

Figure 12.4. EKGs derived from standard limb leads I, II, and III and from a modified Lead II. Leads I and III are less often used by psychophysiologists because they result in a smaller R spike (see first and second channels). Lead II and modified lead II (right collarbone and lower left rib) are more often used by psychophysiologists because these leads produce a pronounced R spike. These four leads were recorded simultaneously from the same person.

ment because the leads are placed on areas that are relatively free of fatty tissue and muscle that may shift during movement. A Lead II or modified Lead II placement is typical in the psychophysiology lab because it generally provides an ECG with a large QRS complex relative to the other components (figure 12.4). One and only one large spike per cycle makes quantification of heart rate much easier.

*Recording Equipment* The QRS complex picked up from the surface of the skin is approximately 1 mV. Often, the signal is amplified, either by a hardware amplifier or by software. In conjunction with the amplification process, the heart signal can be further conditioned by the utilization of filters, as discussed in chapters 3 and 14. When possible, it is better to remove electrical noise from the recording environment, rather than filter the signal to remove the effects of that noise. However, because the highest frequency of interest in the QRS complex is approximately 12 Hz, one can set a high-pass filter at 30–35 Hz, which will both reduce the problem of 60-Hz electrical noise and remove many muscle artifacts. If one wants simply to determine the distance between successive heart beats, one can use an instrument called a cardiotachometer (or cardiotach); this instrument is triggered by the R spike in the QRS complex of each heart beat and gives an output in the form of heart rate that is calculated from the preceding interbeat interval. Heart rate is displayed on the Y axis; with each beat, a new calculation is performed and the new heart rate displayed as a horizontal line on the cardiotach record (see bottom panel of figure 12.5 for an example). A cardiotach display also reveals the oscillations in heart rate referred to previously as RSA. Thus, the figure shows that heart rate increases and decreases in a cyclical fashion that is roughly coincident with respiratory inhalation and exhalation (see figure 12.5). The EKG is generally recorded using an AC amplifier. In this way, one obtains a more stable baseline than would be seen with DC amplification, and this improves visualization of the signal for either computer or cardiotachometer analyses.

*Procedure* What follows is the standard procedure for most psychophysiological experiments in which heart rate is measured. The subject is seated in a comfortable chair and is given information about the experiment. It is a good idea to describe briefly how heart rate is measured and to emphasize that no electricity will be penetrating the subject through the electrodes, but rather that the equipment measures the natural electrical activity of the body without harm. The skin may be cleaned with alcohol on a gauze pad to remove dead skin and skin oils. When standard silver-silver chloride electrodes are used, high conductivity electrode gel is placed in the electrode cup and the electrode is attached to the skin with an adhesive collar or tape. Disposable electrodes, which are commonly used in psychophysiology laboratories, are gelled by the manufacture and are ready to apply.

### Typical Recordings and Common Problems

Figure 12.4 depicts EKGs recorded from the three standard limb leads, along with a modified Lead II placement. Since the voltage of the EKG

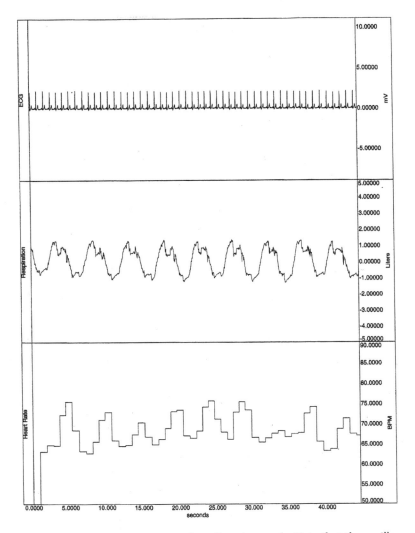

Figure 12.5. EKG, respiration, and cardiotach records. Note that the oscillatory changes in heart rate which can be most easily seen in the bottom channel coincide (albeit with a brief delay) with the respiratory changes in the second channel. These shifts in interbeat interval are much less apparent with the EKG depiction (top channel).

on the surface of the skin is relatively large, there are few problems when recording. The most common problems are 60 Hz interference and movement artifacts. However, these problems can be corrected without great expense by careful choice and preparation of the electrode site and the electrodes. An additional factor that becomes important if the researcher employs a computer or *cardiotachometer* is that the QRS complexes must be easily distinguishable electronically from one another and significantly larger than the P and T waves. As previously noted and as seen in figure 12.4, limb lead II or the modified Lead II usually results in an EKG with these desired characteristics. For additional information about recording heart rate or period, consult Papillo & Shapiro (1990).

## Analysis and Quantification

In the early days of psychophysiological research, the distance between R waves on a paper record was measured with a ruler, and this measure was either converted to heart rate or utilized directly as the measure for analysis. Today most researchers use either a cardiotachometer or a computer for direct analysis of the timing between beats. There are two commonly used measures of cardiac activity: heart rate and *heart period* (or interbeat interval). Heart rate is defined as the number of beats per unit time (usually in minutes). For example, a change in beats per minute may be used to determine the effects of biofeedback training, with the experimenter measuring the number of beats occurring in a 10-min training period relative to the number of beats occurring in a 10-min rest period. Interbeat interval or heart period is determined by measuring the time between R waves (usually in msec). Note that heart rate is simply the reciprocal of heart period. Thus, the timing of the heart beats during 1 min can be reported as either 85 beats/min or 706 ms depending upon the unit of measure used. Because the time units are different for heart period (ms) and heart rate (min), one can convert from one to the other using the following:

$$\text{Heart period (in ms)} = 60000/\text{heart rate (in bpm)}$$
$$\text{Heart rate (in bpm)} = 60000/\text{heart period (in ms)}$$

Often, it has been assumed that the choice of cardiac metric or measure is not important. However, heart rate and heart period are not linearly related to each other. To illustrate this, figure 12.6 shows the relationship between change in activity of the parasympathetic branch and heart rate, and the relationship between parasympathetic change and heart period based on data recorded from dogs. This figure shows that while a given change in activity of an autonomic nerve will result in approximately the same change in heart period for very different baseline heart period values, the same is not true of heart rate. For example, an increase in stimulation frequency of the parasympathetic nerve of 2 Hz results in a change of 70–72 ms in heart period whether the resting (baseline) heart period is 875 ms or 350 ms. However, when the dog's heart is beating at a heart period of 875 ms (or 68.6 bpm) the change in heart rate with a 2 Hz increment in parasympathetic activation is 5.1 bpm, whereas at a baseline heart period of 350 ms, the same 2 Hz change in autonomic input to the heart results in a heart rate change of 29.2 bpm. The same relative linearity also tends to be true for sympathetic

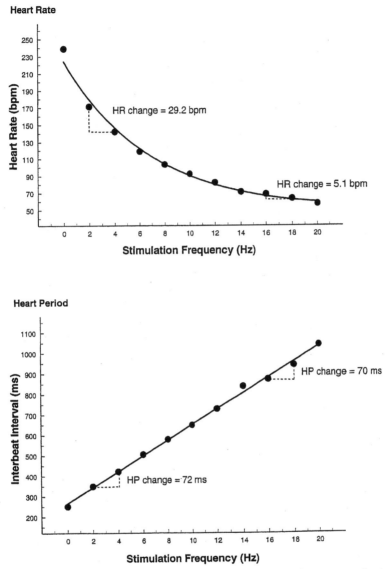

Figure 12.6. Heart period and heart rate as a function of parasympathetic stimulation frequency. Data used for illustration are from a study of vagus nerve (parasympathetic) stimulation in dogs by Parker, Celler, Potter, & Mc-Closkey, 1984. To illustrate the nonlinearity in change scores that would appear as a result of using heart rate rather than heart period, a 2-Hz change in stimulation from 2–4 Hz and from 16–18 Hz are shown for both heart rate and heart period. Lower panel: Note that a 2-Hz increase in stimulation changes heart period a similar amount regardless of whether the stimulation began at 2 Hz or 16 Hz. Upper panel: In contrast, a 2-Hz increase in stimulation of the vagus at 2 Hz changes heart rate by 29.2 bpm, whereas a 2-Hz increase from 16 to 18 Hz only changes heart rate by 5.1 bpm. These data are derived from the same subjects, but the transformation of heart period (which is relatively linear with respect to the parasympathetic input) to heart rate introduces a statistical artifact which alters the *apparent* changes if one were to use heart rate as the metric of cardiac function.

impact on the heart period, and seems to be true for a variety of mammalian species, including humans (Berntson, Cacioppo, & Quigley, 1995; Parker, Celler, Potter, & McCloskey, 1984). Therefore, the amount of cardiac change that the psychophysiologist reports as a result of some environmental or psychological manipulation will differ depending upon the metric chosen to represent the change in cardiac function. Also note that these effects will be most pronounced when baseline autonomic changes are large. Thus, Berntson et al. (1995) have recommended that heart period be used as the metric of choice when (a) the change in cardiac function is likely to be a result of autonomic effects (e.g., for many of the short-term cardiac responses seen in the psychophysiology laboratory), and (b) when the changes in cardiac function are large, where errors due to the nonlinear relationship between autonomic inputs and heart rate will be significant.

In addition to the choice of cardiac measure, one must decide whether to represent cardiac function by computing a mean value for cardiac function over a number of beats (unit of analysis is cardiac time) or over a period of time (unit of analysis is real time). Heart period permits analysis of cardiac function in either cardiac time or real time, whereas heart rate can be represented appropriately only in real time (Berntson et al., 1995; Graham, 1978). As depicted in figure 12.7, heart period can be measured beat by beat or be computed for a particular time period. To compute heart period in real time, it is important to use a weighted averaging procedure so that the average reflects the proportion of time that each beat contributes to the overall average. See figure 12.7 for an example of computing an average weighted heart period or heart rate for a given epoch.

## Cardiac Output

Cardiac output (generally in liters per minute) represents one of the most important cardiodynamic variables because it determines in large part the amount of oxygen and nutrients available to the brain, the heart, and to skeletal muscles that is necessary to sustain life and respond to the internal and external stimuli with which we are constantly confronted. In the past, most measurements of cardiac output were made invasively, which limited their use to clinical settings. However, psychophysiologists now use indirect noninvasive measurements of cardiac output. The two noninvasive procedures most commonly used in the laboratory are impedance cardiography (ZCG) and combined-Doppler ultrasound. The combined-Doppler ultrasound procedure, however is currently too expensive to be found in many psychophysiological labs; this has made impedance cardiography the current method of choice. Impedance cardiography is a technique that provides a measure of changes

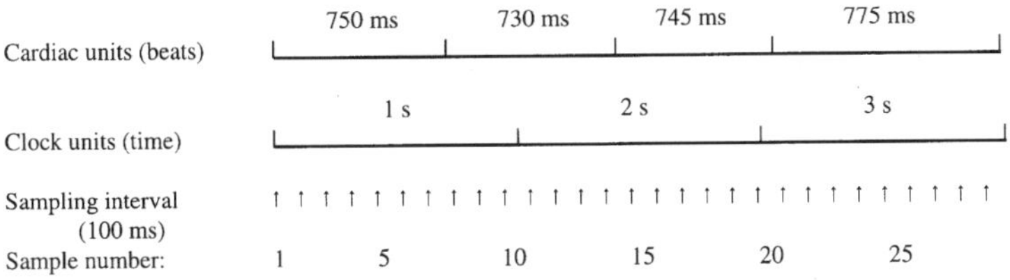

| | 750 ms | 730 ms | 745 ms | 775 ms |
|---|---|---|---|---|
| Cardiac units (beats) | | | | |

| | 1 s | 2 s | 3 s |
|---|---|---|---|
| Clock units (time) | | | |

Sampling interval
(100 ms)

↑ ↑ ↑ ↑ ↑ ↑ ↑ ↑ ↑ ↑ ↑ ↑ ↑ ↑ ↑ ↑ ↑ ↑ ↑ ↑ ↑ ↑ ↑ ↑ ↑ ↑ ↑ ↑ ↑ ↑ ↑ ↑

| Sample number: | 1 | 5 | 10 | 15 | 20 | 25 |
|---|---|---|---|---|---|---|

**Averages**:

| Second 1: | Sample 1 | 750 ms | Sample 6 | 750 ms |
|---|---|---|---|---|
| | Sample 2 | 750 ms | Sample 7 | 750 ms |
| | Sample 3 | 750 ms | Sample 8 | 730 ms |
| | Sample 4 | 750 ms | Sample 9 | 730 ms |
| | Sample 5 | 750 ms | Sample 10 | <u>730 ms</u> |
| | | | | 7440 ms/10 samples |

**Weighted Average Heart Period**:

Take the sum of the interbeat intervals for all samples in the time period ÷ # of samples.

Examples:

**Second 1**:

Weighted HP = (750 ms X 7 samples) + (730 X 3 samples) ÷ 10 samples = 7440 ÷ 10 = 744 ms/beat

**Seconds 1-3**:

Weighted HP = (750 ms X 7 samples) + (730 ms X 7 samples) + (745 ms X 6 samples) + (775 X 9 samples)
   ÷ 29 samples = (5250 + 5110 + 4470 + 6975) ÷ 29 = 751.9 ms/beat

**Weighted Average Heart Rate**:

Take the inverse of the weighted average HP and convert to beats/min.

Example:

**Second 1**:
$$\text{Weighted HR} = \left( \frac{744\ \text{ms X}\ 1\ \text{s X}\ 1\ \text{min}}{\text{beat X}\ 1000\ \text{ms X}\ 60\ \text{s}} \right)^{-1} = 60000 \div 744 = 80.6\ \text{beats/min (or bpm)}$$

Figure 12.7. Calculation of weighted average heart period and heart rate. The upper part of the figure shows a series of four intervals representing four interbeat intervals of 750, 730, 745, and 775 ms, respectively. The next part of the figure depicts a clock running along with the interbeat intervals. In this case, the clock began timing as the first interbeat interval began. Sampling of a value by the computer is shown in the next line, with a sample of the data taken at each 100 ms interval beginning with the start of the clock and time zero. Calculations are shown for deriving both weighted heart period (examples of a 1-s and 3-s weighted average) and for weighted heart rate (example of a 1-s weighted average).

in blood flow in the thorax. From those changes one can derive measures of stroke volume. Recall that cardiac output is the product of heart rate and stroke volume. Thus, combining measures from the EKG and the impedance cardiogram, one can derive a noninvasive estimate of cardiac output. It appears that cardiac output derived from impedance cardiography is likely to be a biased estimate of the true absolute cardiac output, but the relative measures of changes in cardiac output are valid. For a review of various methods for measuring cardiac output, including noninvasive measures, see Ehlers, Mylrea, Waterson, and Calkins (1986). For more information on impedance cardiography see Sherwood et al. (1990), and Miller and Horvath (1978).

# Blood Pressure

Since the seventeenth century, scientists have had some understanding of the function of the circulatory system, but it was not until 1733 that blood pressure was first measured. Before that time, it was believed that blood circulation was maintained at each heart beat by a force of 100,000 pounds. Steven Hales, a scientist and Anglican priest, was the first person to measure blood pressure in animals and dispel what he considered to be "unsatisfactory conjectures." Hales inserted a flexible tube, or cannula, into an artery of a horse which was, in turn, connected to a long glass tube open at one end. With each beat of the horse's heart, the blood would rise or fall within the tube, thus yielding a measure of the animal's blood pressure (Cohen, 1976). An instrument is still in use for animal research based on the same principle as Hales's device. A refinement of this direct method still remains the most accurate measure of human blood pressure, although there is only a limited number of situations (e.g., surgery) where it can be applied.

Before considering methods of measuring blood pressure, let us review the pumping of the heart as it relates to pressure. It was previously stated that blood low in oxygen returns to the right side of the heart from the body, enters the right atrium, then flows into the right ventricle and from there is pumped into the lungs. Following this, the oxygenated blood returns to the heart through the left atrium and then into the left ventricle for distribution throughout the body. It is the contraction of the left ventricle that produces the necessary pressure to move the blood throughout the body. Sufficient pressure must be generated to push blood through the arteries, capillaries, and veins. The larger arteries and veins require smaller differences in pressure across the length of the vessel for blood flow than do the small vessels where resistance to flow will be relatively high.

The maximal, or *systolic*, blood pressure occurs when the ventricle of the heart contracts. Following the period of cardiac contraction, there is relaxation (diastole) of the ventricle, during which blood pressure is at a minimum; a measurement at this time yields *diastolic* pressure. In general, diastolic pressure varies mostly with peripheral resistance, whereas systolic pressure is related to both peripheral resistance and stroke volume. Blood pressure is reported as systolic pressure over diastolic pressure. The standard unit of measurement is millimeters of mercury, abbreviated as "mmHg." The typical blood pressure of a healthy college student is 120/80 mmHg, although various factors, such as age, diet, posture, and weight, are important.

Pulse pressure is the pressure difference between systolic and diastolic pressures. In the case of the typical college student, the pulse pressure would be about 40 mmHg (120 − 80 = 40). Some researchers calculate the *mean arterial pressure*, which is generally defined as diastolic pressure plus 1/3 pulse pressure.

### Recording Procedure

In clinical practice, both direct and indirect measures of blood pressure are used. The direct measure uses a catheter that is inserted into a vessel or heart cavity. The direct method is infrequently used in psychophysiological research and the interested reader should consult a medically oriented text (e.g., Guyton & Hall, 1996), for more details. For additional information about non-invasive recording of blood pressure consult Papillo and Shapiro (1990).

*Indirect Measurement*    The most common indirect measure of blood pressure employs a *sphygmomanometer*. This device, commonly found in physicians' offices, consists of a pressure cuff connected to a tube containing mercury. The present method dates back to the beginning of this century and was introduced by Korotkoff. The following is a step-by-step procedure for determining both systolic and diastolic blood pressure.

The blood pressure cuff is placed on the upper arm, with a stethoscope over the brachial artery and just below the cuff (figure 12.8). When the cuff is inflated to a pressure sufficient to cut off all arterial blood flow, no sound is heard through the stethoscope. As the pressure in the cuff is slowly reduced, the so-called Korotkoff sounds (tapping sounds) appear. The cuff pressure at which the first sound is heard is read as systolic pressure and is referred to as the start of phase I. As the pressure in the cuff continues to decrease, the sounds take on a murmuring quality (phase II) and then become clearer and louder (phase III). Following this, Korotkoff sounds become muffled (phase IV). This lasts for the next 5 to 6 mmHg fall in pressure, until the sounds disappear completely (phase V). In general medical practice and typically in the psychophysiology laboratory, the pressure at phase V is considered the diastolic blood pressure. Certain methodological and experimental problems exist in recording blood pressure. First, blood pressure is not static, even though our use of absolute numbers might lead us to believe otherwise. Rather, as pointed out more than 200 years ago by Hales, there is a natural variation in the system. A normal individual's blood pressure can vary as much as 30 mmHg during a 1-min recording using a direct blood pressure technique (Tursky, 1974).

When using a sphygmomanometer to obtain indirect blood pressure, a number of factors must be taken into account. First, there are factors related to the technique itself. Repeated measurements within a short period will produce (through the inflation and deflation of the pressure cuff) temporary tissue changes that result in different blood pressure readings. Second, there are factors related to the instrument being used. Most

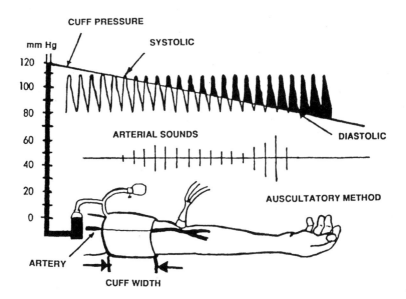

Figure 12.8. Auscultatory method for measuring blood pressure. The auscultatory method relies on the changes in sounds in a microphone located over the artery, which has been briefly occluded. First, the occluding cuff is pumped full of air to a relatively high pressure (above systolic pressure). Then, air is gradually bled from the cuff. The blood pressure at which the first arterial sounds appear is read as the systolic blood pressure. Diastolic pressure is typically read as the pressure in the cuff when the last arterial sound disappears. When using this method, mean arterial pressure is calculated from the systolic and diastolic pressures (see text for the formula). Figure is from L. A. Geddes, 1991, *Handbook of blood pressure measurement*, Clifton, NJ: Humana Press.

notably, the size of the cuff can change the blood pressure recorded. To determine the appropriate cuff size, the circumference of the upper arm is first determined. The cuff width should be at least 40% of arm circumference, and the cuff length should be at least 80% of the circumference (Bailey & Bauer, 1993). In addition, the closed pressure system of the instrument must be free of all leaks (e.g., of air or mercury) in order for the measurements to be valid. Finally, blood pressure can vary due to factors related to the person's situation. For example, several investigators have found higher blood pressure readings when they are taken in a clinical setting than when they are taken during a normal day (a phenomenon known as "white-coat hypertension"). Similarly, a subject coming for a psychophysiological experiment may initially experience anxiety or fear concerning the situation or the equipment, and thus demonstrate blood pressures that differ from normal readings before the experiment has even begun. Another set of factors that also should be considered is related to individual differences in the skills of the experimenter. That is, since the presence and absence of Korotkoff sounds require a judgment on the part of the experimenter, the precision with which the recording is made and the skill of the experimenter must also be considered.

*Automated Indirect Measurement*   Automated devices for measuring blood pressure are available and can be utilized with a polygraph or computer, or the measurements can simply be read from a visual display on the front panel of the instrument. These devices employ either a microphone in the cuff (auscultatory method) or a pressure transducer in the cuff (oscillometric method). The auscultatory method utilizes Korotkoff sounds transduced by the microphone in the cuff in the same way as would be done by a human observer using a manual recording system. Systolic pressure is taken to be that point at which the first Korotkoff sound appears on the polygraph record and diastolic pressure the level at which the last sound appears. With this method, it is easier to accurately determine systolic than diastolic pressure. The oscillometric method utilizes oscillations in pressure in the cuff to determine systolic, diastolic, and mean arterial pressure (Borow & Newberger, 1982). With this method, following inflation of the cuff to a pressure above the systolic pressure, the cuff is deflated in steps. The systolic pressure is taken as the pressure when the oscillations in the cuff first begin to get larger, the mean arterial pressure is taken as the point when the cuff oscillations are maximal in size, and the diastolic pressure is taken as the point when the cuff pressure oscillations no longer become smaller in amplitude (see figure 12.9).

A major problem with both the manual and automated procedures for obtaining indirect measures of blood pressure is that a cuff must be inflated and deflated. This is sometimes a stronger stimulus for the subject than the independent variable and it also limits the number of readings that can be taken in a given session. The development of continuous blood pressure recording devices removes the need for repeated cuff inflations. These devices are in use in many psychophysiology labs, but the most affordable devices were removed from the market. Currently, several relatively expensive beat-to-beat recording devices are available, and it is likely that less expensive devices will reappear on the market. The two most commonly used devices for the psychophysiological lab use either arterial tonometry or vascular unloading (also known as the method of Peñáz). Blood pressure is measured using the arterial tonometry method by placing a sensor over an artery that overlies bone. Slight pressure is applied to the artery, and the pressure in the partially flattened artery is recorded as the arterial pressure. The most common site for tonometric measurements is the radial artery at the wrist. Care must be taken that the sensor is placed directly over the artery and that no movement of the artery or sensor takes place during the recording session (Kemmotsu, Ueda, Otsuka, Yamamura, Winter, & Eckerle, 1991). The vascular un-

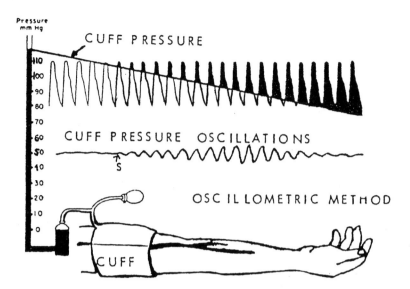

Figure 12.9. Oscillometric method for measuring blood pressure. The oscillometric method relies on the transduction of oscillations in the cuff pressure to derive blood pressure. The occluding cuff is pumped full of air to a relatively high pressure (above systolic pressure). Then, air is gradually bled from the cuff. Oscillations in the pressure inside the cuff are used to mark systolic, mean arterial, and diastolic pressures. Systolic pressure is determined when pressure oscillations first appear as the pressure in the occluding cuff is bled off. Mean arterial pressure is taken as the point where the pressure oscillations are maximal in size, and diastolic pressure is taken as the point when the last pressure oscillations in the cuff disappear. Figure is from L. A. Geddes, 1991, *Handbook of blood pressure measurement*, Clifton, NJ: Humana Press.

loading method typically uses a cuff on the finger to clamp the vascular volume of the finger at a specific level which is maintained from beat to beat. The volume is measured using a plethysmographic device, which reflects changes in blood volume beneath the sensor (see section on blood volume); then, using a servo-control system, changes are made in the pressure within the finger cuff, and the artery is returned to its previous volume. The amount of pressure change needed in the finger cuff to reestablish the volume in the artery is a function of the arterial pressure underlying the cuff (Shapiro et al., 1996).

### Analysis and Quantification

The measurement and quantification of blood pressure data are related and often limited to the particular measuring device used. For example, even when the cuff method is automated, it is not recommended that the experimenter take more than one reading per minute (Shapiro et al.,

1996). Beat-to-beat recordings permit blood pressure determinations for each beat, which will result in a greater reliability of measurements. Because of the variability in blood pressure that was noted previously, it is recommended that multiple blood pressure readings taken from a recording epoch be averaged to provide a more stable estimate of the blood pressure for that epoch.

## Blood Volume and Flow

Many individuals have experienced vasomotor changes, such as cold feet and hands, while waiting for someone special or preparing to take an important examination; others have experienced a flushing or blushing during emotional arousal. As was mentioned earlier in this chapter, changes in blood volume may be produced by either a decrease or an increase in sympathetic nervous system activity.

The two most commonly used vasomotor measures in psychophysiological research are blood volume and pulse volume. Blood volume recordings reflect relatively slow changes (i.e., changes in tonic level) in the amount of blood in an arm, leg, finger, or toe. Pulse volume is a phasic measure of the pulsatile change in blood flow related both to the pumping action of the heart and to the vasodilation and constriction of vessels in the periphery. Thus, pulse volume is a measure of the amplitude of individual pulses.

### Recording Procedure

The most common measure of blood volume used in psychophysiological laboratories today is that of *plethysmography*. The term "plethysmography" comes from a Greek word that can be translated as "enlargement" or "fullness." Technically, a plethysmograph is a device for measuring the change in volume of a given structure such as an arm, leg, finger, or even the entire body. Thus, a true plethysmograph would consist of a sealed chamber in which the arm, leg, or other structure is placed. Since the chamber is sealed, any change in the volume within the chamber would cause a recordable pressure change.

Although there are a variety of techniques for measuring blood volume and pulse volume, the three most commonly used are (1) photoelectric changes, (2) impedance changes, and (3) volume changes recorded with a strain gauge.

*Photoelectric Plethysmography* By far the most popular plethysmographic technique employs a photocell placed over an area of tissue perfused with blood. There are two basic variations of this method: a light source can pass through the tissue segment (transillumined) or bounce off the tissue (backscattered). The amount of light that passes through or is reflected back is received by a photoelectric transducer and converted into electrical energy for recording. The light source produces light in the infrared range (7000–9000 Å). Since electromagnetic radiation in this frequency is scattered by blood, the output of a photodetector may be considered related to the amount of blood within the region (Jennings, Tahmoush, & Redmond, 1980; Tursky & Jamner, 1982). Currently, most plethysmographic devices utilize either a light-emitting diode (LED) or a phototransistor that has minimal effects on the underlying skin and blood vessels so that the device does not alter the tissue being recorded from.

If the light is transmitted through the tissue to a photodetector on the other side, only a limited number of sites are convenient (e.g., the earlobe). However, as demonstrated by Stern (1974), blood flow changes in the earlobe are not particularly responsive to typical laboratory tasks and stressors such as viewing slides of auto accidents or nudes, or performing mental arithmetic. With the backscattered photoelectric plethysmographic technique, the light source and the photodetector are both located on the same side of the tissue and thus can be placed almost anywhere on the body. The backscattered photoplethysmograph is more sensitive to the vascular fluctuations occurring close to the surface of the skin, whereas the transillumined photoplethysmograph is sensitive to both skin and deeper tissue vascular changes. For an example of a recent study employing photoplethysmography, see Spence, Shapiro, and Zaidel (1996).

*Impedance Plethysmography*   In chapter 10, impedance was mentioned as a method of recording respiration. It can also be used to record blood volume changes. One of the major advantages of the impedance method is that it is not prone to artifacts caused by EKG, EMG, and other electrical activity observed at the surface of the skin. The procedure employs two electrodes on the skin through which a high-frequency alternating current is passed. Since human tissue is a good conductor of alternating current, and since changes in the amount of blood volume in a given tissue segment produce changes in electrical impedance, it is possible to infer indirectly the change of blood volume taking place. This technique is the same as impedance cardiography in which the segment of interest is the torso. For a recent study using impedance plethysmography in body segments other than the torso, see White and Montgomery (1996).

*Strain Gauge Plethysmography*   Previously we discussed the application of strain gauges for measuring changes in respiration. Using the same principle, strain gauges may also be used to measure changes in blood volume and pulse volume. The strain gauge is placed around the finger, toe, or other body segment; changes in resistance or voltage of the strain gauge can be considered an indirect measurement of blood volume changes. The strain gauge is well suited for application on the penis where other devices work less well. Indeed, use of the penile strain gauge has become especially important in studies of male responses to erotic stimuli and studies of treatments for sex offenders (see Farrall, 1992, for a discussion of the use of the penile plethysmograph for assessing sexual arousal).

*Venous Occlusion Plethysmography*   Venous occlusion plethysmography is a recording technique for measuring changes in blood flow to segments of the limbs. This technique generally requires two cuffs, one placed distal to the limb segment of interest, and one placed proximal to the limb segment. The distal cuff is inflated to a pressure above the systolic arterial pressure in order to prevent blood flow into and out of the distal limb segment. The proximal cuff is inflated to a pressure level that is sufficient to eliminate venous flow from the limb segment, but which does not prevent arterial flow into the segment. A strain gauge is placed around the limb segment being measured, and the change in limb circumference per unit of time is used to infer the rate of blood flow into the segment. The advantage of this method is that arterial blood flow into the isolated limb segment can be measured independent of other possible sources of blood flow change (e.g., venous flow). One obvious limitation of the venous occlusion technique is that measurements cannot be taken continuously; even at very short intervals, numbness or pain in the limb can result. In addition, measurements can be altered by movement of the limb. For a recent example of the use of the venous occlusion plethysmographic technique, see Lindqvist, Melcher, and Hjemdahl (1997).

### Typical Recordings and Common Problems

Figure 12.10 shows two typical recordings of vasomotor activity: blood volume and pulse volume. As noted previously, the blood volume measure represents the relatively slow changes of blood in a particular structure, such as an arm or a leg. Measurements of blood volume are made using a DC amplifier connected to an appropriate preamplifier and to whatever type of transducer is used. In figure 12.10, a photoelectric cell sensed the blood volume changes. Likewise, pulse volume changes were recorded with a photoelectric cell on the finger, except that the amplifier used was AC coupled. Recall that AC coupling removes some of the slower frequency shifts in the DC coupled signal. Pulse volume recordings reflect the changes in blood flow to an area with each beat of the heart.

Jennings, Tahmoush, and Redmond (1980) and Tursky and Jamner (1982) reviewed many of the factors that influence vasomotor changes and discussed problems of interpretation from the indirect measures that have been described here. For example, changes in room temperature

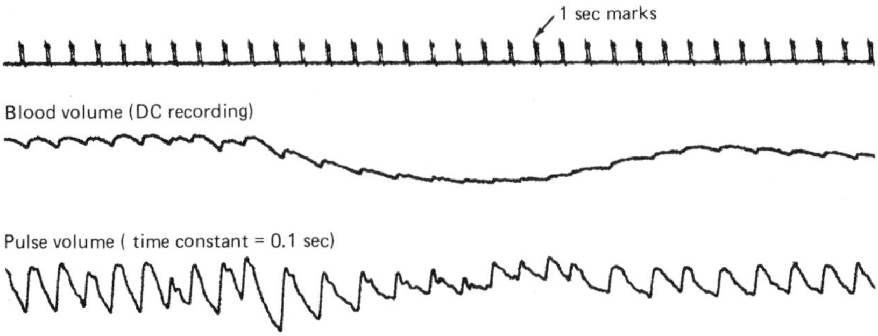

Figure 12.10. Blood volume and pulse volume recorded simultaneously. Note that the blood volume was DC coupled whereas the pulse volume was AC coupled. AC coupling removes the slow drift.

during a study from one day to the next could result in differential results unrelated to the experimental situation, especially using the measure of pulse volume. Another problem is related to the wide variation in skin characteristics (e.g., location of vessels), which makes absolute comparisons between subjects impossible. Even within the same subject, difficulty in precise placement of the transducer makes comparisons only relative. It should also be pointed out that since different areas of the body contain differential distributions of muscles and blood vessels, it is difficult to compare results between studies when varying transducer sites are used. Finally, one must remember that blood flow is a complex function of pressure in the vasculature, the radius of the blood vessels, and the viscosity of the blood. Moreover, flow changes may occur in a given segment by means of arterial or venous flow changes either into or out of the segment of interest. Thus, one must be cautious in making interpretations about the mechanisms underlying indirectly measured blood flow changes.

## Analysis and Quantification

Because of the relative nature of the vasomotor measurements performed by most psychophysiologists, experimenters typically examine changes for each participant from a baseline period and compare this to the experimental or treatment period. The change between baseline and treatment is generally expressed as a percentage. The magnitude of an individual pulse is determined by simply measuring the difference between the lowest point and the peak and a computer can be programmed to detect the minimum and maximum points. Some researchers have used an integrating coupler to perform a similar function. Because integration of a curve represents the area under the curve, this may also represent relative pulse volume changes.

As always in psychophysiology, new methodological advances will likely enhance our ability to measure a greater number and variety of hemodynamic variables, which will permit a more comprehensive picture of the complexities of the cardiovascular system.

*References*

Anderson, E. A., & Mark, A. L. (1989). Microneurographic measurement of sympathetic nerve activity in humans. In N. Schneiderman, S. M. Weiss, and P. G. Kaufmann (Eds.), *Handbook of research methods in cardiovascular behavioral medicine* (pp. 107–115). New York: Plenum.

Anderson, E. A., Wallin, B. G., & Mark, A. L. (1987). Dissociation of sympathetic nerve activity to arm and leg during mental stress. *Hypertension, 9*, III-114–III-119.

Bailey, R. H. & Bauer, J. H. (1993). A review of common errors in the indirect measurement of blood pressure: Sphygmomanometry. *Archives of Internal Medicine, 153*, 2741–2748.

Berntson, G. G., Bigger, J. T., Eckberg, D. L., Grossman, P., Kaufmann, P. G., Malik, M., Nagaraja, H. N., Porges, S. W., Saul, J. P., Stone, P. H., & van der Molen, M. W. (1997). Heart rate variability: Origins, methods and interpretive caveats. *Psychophysiology, 34*, 623–648.

Berntson, G. G., Cacioppo, J. T., Binkley, P. F., Uchino, B. N., Quigley, K. S., & Fieldstone, A. (1994). Autonomic cardiac control. III. Psychological stress and cardiac response in autonomic space as revealed by pharmacological blockades. *Psychophysiology, 31*, 599–608.

Berntson, G. G., Cacioppo, J. T., & Quigley, K. S. (1991). Autonomic determinism: The modes of autonomic control, the doctrine of autonomic space, and the laws of autonomic constraint. *Psychological Review, 98*, 459–487.

Berntson, G. G., Cacioppo, J. T., & Quigley, K. S. (1993). Respiratory sinus arrhythmia: Autonomic origins, physiological mechanisms, and psychophysiological implications. *Psychophysiology, 30*, 183–196.

Berntson, G. G., Cacioppo, J. T., & Quigley, K. S. (1995). The metrics of cardiac chronotropism: Biometric perspectives. *Psychophysiology, 32*, 162–171.

Borow, K. M., & Newberger, J. W. (1982). Noninvasive estimation of central aortic pressure using the oscillometric method for analyzing systemic artery pulsatile blood flow: Comparative study of indirect systolic, diastolic, and mean brachial pressure with simultaneous direct ascending aortic pressure measurements. *American Heart Journal, 103*, 879–886.

Cohen, I. B. (1976). Steven Hales. *Scientific American, 234*, 98–107.

Ehlers, K. C., Mylrea, K. C., Waterson, C. K., & Calkins, J. M. (1986). Cardiac output measurements: A review of current techniques and research. *Annals of Biomedical Engineering, 14*, 219–239.

Farrall, W. R. (1992). Instrumentation and methodological issues in the assessment of sexual arousal. In W. O'Donohue & J. H. Geer (Eds.), *The sexual abuse of children: Clinical issues, Vol. 2*. Hillsdale, NJ: Erlbaum.

Geddes, L. A. (1991). *Handbook of blood pressure measurement*. Clifton, NJ: Humana.

Graham, F. K. (1978). Constraints on measuring heart rate and period sequentially through real and cardiac time. *Psychophysiology, 15,* 492–495.

Green, J. F. (1987). *Fundamental cardiovascular and pulmonary physiology* (2nd ed.). Philadelphia: Lea & Fibiger.

Grossman, P., van Beek, J., & Wientjes, C. (1990). A comparison of three quantification methods for estimation of respiratory sinus arrhythmia. *Psychophysiology, 27,* 702–714.

Guyton, A. C., & Hall, J. E. (1996). *Textbook of medical physiology.* Philadelphia: Saunders.

Jennings, J. R., Tahmoush, A. J., & Redmond, D. P. (1980). Non-invasive measurement of peripheral vascular activity. In I. Martin & P. H. Venables (Eds.), *Techniques in psychophysiology* (pp. 69–137). New York: John Wiley.

Kemmotsu, O., Ueda, M., Otsuka, H., Yamamura, T., Winter, D. C., & Eckerle, J. S. (1991). Arterial tonometry for noninvasive, continuous blood pressure monitoring during anesthesia. *Anesthesiology, 75,* 333–340.

Khachaturian, Z. S., Kerr, J. Kruger, R., & Schachter, J. (1972). A methodological note: Comparison between period and rate data in studies of cardiac function. *Psychophysiology, 9,* 539–545.

Lacey, J. T. (1967). Somatic response patterning and stress: Some revision of activation theory. In M. H. Appley and R. Trumbull (Eds.), *Psychological Stress* (pp. 14–37). New York: Appleton Century Crofts.

Lacey, J. I., Kagan, J., Lacey, B. C., & Moss, H. A. (1963). The visceral level: Situational determinants and behavioral correlates of autonomic response patterns. In P. H. Knapp (Ed.), *Expression of the emotions in man* (pp. 161–196). New York: International Universities Press.

Lacey, J. I., & Lacey, B. C. (1980). The specific role of heart rate in sensorimotor integration. In R. F. Thompson, L. H. Hicks, & V. B. Shvyrkov (Eds.), *Neural mechanisms of goal-directed behavior and learning* (pp. 495–509). New York: Academic Press.

Lindqvist, M., Melcher, A., & Hjemdahl, P. (1997). Attenuation of forearm vasodilator responses to mental stress by regional beta-blockade, but not by atropine. *Acta Physiologica Scandinavica, 161,* 135–140.

Miller, J. C., & Horvath, S. M. (1978). Impedance cardiography. *Psychophysiology, 15,* 80–91.

Newlin, D. B., & Levenson, R. W. (1979). Pre-ejection period: Measuring beta-adrenergic influences on the heart. *Psychophysiology, 16,* 546–553.

Obrist, P. (1981). Cardiac-somatic uncoupling. In P. A. Obrist (Ed.), *Cardiovascular psychophysiology: A perspective* (pp. 83–118). New York: Plenum.

Obrist, P. (1982). Cardiac-behavioral interactions: A critical appraisal. In J. T. Cacioppo and R. E. Petty (Eds.), *Perspectives in cardiovascular psychophysiology* (pp. 265–295). New York: Guilford.

Obrist, P. A., Webb, R. A., Sutterer, J. R., & Howard, J. L. (1970). Cardiac deceleration and reaction time: An evaluation of two hypotheses. *Psychophysiology, 6,* 695–706.

Papillo, J. F., & Shapiro, D. (1990). The cardiovascular system. In J. T. Cacioppo and L. G. Tassinary (Eds.), *Principles of psychophysiology: Physical, social, and inferential elements* (pp. 456–512). New York: Cambridge University Press.

Parker, P., Celler, B. G., Potter, E. K., & McCloskey, D. I. (1984). Vagal stimulation and cardiac slowing. *Journal of the Autonomic Nervous System, 11,* 2226–231.

Philips, R., & Feeney, M. (1973). *Cardiac rhythms.* Philadelphia: Saunders.

Porges, S. W. (1986). Respiratory sinus arrhythmia: Physiological basis, quantitative methods, and clinical implications. In P. Grossman, K. Janssen, & D. Vaitl (Eds.), *Cardiorespiratory and cardiosomatic psychophysiology* (pp. 101–115). New York: Plenum.

Porges, S. W., & Bohrer, R. E. (1990). The analysis of periodic processes in psychophysiological research. In J. T. Cacioppo & L. G. Tassinary (Eds.), *Principles of psychophysiology: Physical, social, and inferential elements* (pp. 708–753). New York: Cambridge University Press.

Rothschuh, K. E. (1973). *History of Physiology.* (G. B. Risse, Trans.) Huntington, NY: Krieger. (Original work published 1972)

Shapiro, D., Jamner, L. D., Lane, J. D., Light, K. C., Myrtek, M., Sawada, Y., & Steptoe, A. (1996). Blood pressure publication guidelines. *Psychophysiology, 33,* 1–12.

Sherwood, A., Allen, M. T., Fahrenberg, J., Kelsey, R. M., Lovallo, W. R., & van Doornen, L. J. P. (1990). Methodological guidelines for impedance cardiography. *Psychophysiology, 27,* 1–23.

Spence, S., Shapiro, D., & Zaidel, E. (1996). The role of the right hemisphere in the physiological and cognitive components of emotional processing. *Psychophysiology, 33,* 112–122.

Stern, R. M. (1974). Ear lobe photoplethysmography. *Psychophysiology, 11,* 73–75.

Turner, J. R. (1994). Cardiac-metabolic dissociation: Additional heart rates during psychological stress. In *Cardiovascular reactivity and stress: Patterns of physiological response* (pp. 91–107). New York: Plenum Press.

Tursky, B. (1974). The indirect recording of blood pressure. In P. A. Obrist, A. H. Black, J. Brener, & L. V. DiCara (Eds.), *Cardiovascular psychophysiology* (pp. 93–105). Chicago: Aldine.

Tursky, B., & Jamner, L. D. (1982). Measurement of cardiovascular functioning. In J. T. Cacioppo R. E. Petty (Eds.), *Perspectives in cardiovascular psychophysiology* (pp. 19–92). New York: Guilford.

White, D. D., & Montgomery, L. D. (1996). Pelvic pooling of men and women during lower body negative pressure. *Aviation Space, and Environmental Medicine, 67,* 555–559.

Wientjes, C. J. E. (1992). Respiration in psychophysiology: Methods and applications. *Biological Psychology, 34,* 179–203.

# 13

## Skin

*Electrodermal Activity*

---

Electrodermal recording continues stoutly to provide useful data in spite of being abused by measurement techniques which range from the arbitrary to the positively weird.

(Lykken and Venables, 1971, p. 656)

*Electrodermal activity* (EDA) has been recorded in thousands of psychophysiological studies. Why is this such a popular measure? Many who record EDA today share the basic belief expressed by Carl Jung in 1907 and also by present-day lie detector operators that verbal responses do not tell all, but that EDA does reveal the secrets of "mental life." Neumann and Blanton (1970), in a fascinating history of early EDA research which was referred to in chapter 1, noted the "mind-reading" view of EDA that was made popular by Jung's word-association experiments. Peterson (1907), a student of Jung, described the experiments as follows: "It is like fishing in the sea of the unconscious, and the fish that likes the bait best jumps to the hook. . . . Every stimulus accompanied by an emotion produced a deviation of the galvanometer to a degree of direct proportion to the liveliness and actuality of the emotion aroused" (p. 805).

Today we think of EDA as a measure of the state of the organism's interaction with its environment. EDA reflects not only emotional responding; it is also elicited by cognitive activity (e.g., Siddle, 1991). Edelberg (1972) reminded us that the skin has a special significance because it both receives outside information and responds to signals from within. He further states, "We can listen in on such signals by taking advantage of the fact that their arrival at the skin is heralded by measurable electrified changes that we call electrodermal activity" (p. 368). If we think of our skin as a giant receptor separating us from the rest of the world, is it any wonder that responses obtained from it would be of interest to psychologists?

From an evolutionary standpoint, the survival value of EDA is a perplexing issue and one not easily studied. Why do the palms of our hands and the bottoms of our feet sweat when we are anxious? Darrow suggested (1933) that this response has persisted through evolution because it aids grasping—for example, grasping of vines in flight, grasping of clubs when fighting, grasping of tennis rackets, and so on. Edelberg (1973) has written about the relationship of changes in the electrical activity of the skin to survival functions such as locomotion, manipulation, and defense.

## Terminology

The terms used to describe EDA have changed over the years. The term used at the turn of the nineteenth century was "psychogalvanic reflex." Later the term "galvanic skin response" was used. Today most psychophysiologists favor the term electrodermal activity.

The electrical activity of the skin can be measured in two ways. First, a small current can be passed through the skin from an external source and the resistance to the passage of current then measured. This technique was first used by Feré in 1888 and is referred to as the exosomatic method. The second method, the endosomatic technique, was first used by Tarchanoff in 1889; it measures the electrical activity at the surface of the skin, with no externally imposed current. The exosomatic method has been modified today into the measurement of *skin conductance* (SC), the reciprocal of skin resistance. The endosomatic method is still used to measure skin potential (SP), but skin conductance recording is used today by most researchers.

When describing electrodermal activity, one can discuss basal activity (tonic) versus the response to a stimulus (phasic) (see chapter 4). When referring to tonic electrodermal activity, the convention is to use the word level (L); when discussing phasic activity, the convention is to use the word response (R). Therefore, the four common descriptions of electrodermal activity are as follows:

*skin conductance level* (SCL);

*skin conductance response* (SCR);

*skin potential level* (SPL);

*skin potential response* (SPR).

As stated in chapter 4, psychophysiological recordings show a third type of activity in addition to tonic and phasic activity: spontaneous or nonspecific activity. Electrodermal activity is no exception. Spontaneous electrodermal activity appears in records obtained using both the SC and SP techniques.

Table 13.1 summarizes the various skin conductance measures used by researchers and provides some expected values; this information is from Dawson, Schell, and Filion (1990). The reader is referred to their chapter for a more detailed discussion of electrodermal activity.

Figure 13.1 shows a simultaneous recording of SC and SP. The SPR is usually biphasic, with the negative component followed by the positive component. In some cases SPR is uniphasic negative. The latency of SCR and the negative phase of SPR are usually between 1.0 and 3.0 s. Note that SCL and SPL changed during the few seconds of this recording. These relatively slow or gradual changes in SCL and SPL are not considered to be examples of SCR or SPR. The latter terms are reserved for the more

**Table 13.1** Electrodermal Measures, Definitions, and Typical Values

| Measure | Definition | Typical Values |
|---|---|---|
| Skin conductance level (SCL) | Tonic level of electrical conductivity of skin | 2–20 *microsiemens* (μS) |
| Change in SCL | Gradual changes in SCL measured at two or more points in time | 1–3 μS |
| Frequency of NS-SCRs | Number of SCRs in absence of identifiable eliciting stimulus | 1–3 per min |
| ER-SCR amplitude | Phasic increase in conductance shortly following stimulus onset | 0.2–1.0 μS |
| ER-SCR latency | Temporal interval between stimulus onset and SCR initiation | 1–3 s |
| ER-SCR rise time | Temporal interval between SCR initiation and SCR peak | 1–3 s |
| ER-SCR half recovery time | Temporal interval between SCR peak and point of 50% recovery of SCR amplitude | 2–10 s |
| ER-SCR habituation (trials to habituation) | Number of stimulus presentations before two or three trials with no response | 2–8 stimulus presentations |
| ER-SCR habituation (slope) | Rate of change of ER-SCR amplitude | 0.01–0.5 μS per trial |

*Source:* From M. Dawson, A. Schell, and D. Filion, 1990, "The electrodermal system." In J. T. Cacioppo and L. G. Tassinary (Eds.), *Principles of psychophysiology,* Cambridge: Cambridge University Press. Reprinted by permission.

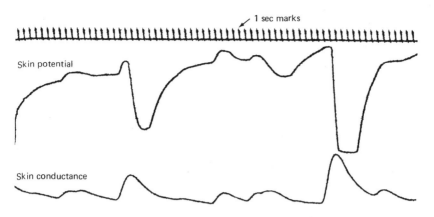

1 sec marks

Skin potential

Skin conductance

Figure 13.1. A simultaneous recording of skin potential and skin conductance.

rapid responses to stimuli, which show the latency and shape of the responses in figure 13.1.

## Physiological Basis

We turn now to a brief summary of what is known about the underlying physiological mechanisms of electrodermal activity. For additional information, consult Dawson, Schell, and Filion (1990) or Boucsein (1992).

We still do not know a great deal about the complex relationship of the central nervous system to EDA. Boucsein (1992) has proposed a two-component model of this relationship. According to Boucsein, there are two separate portions of the central nervous system that are involved in the control of EDA activity: an ipsilateral system—the hypothalamus, anterior thalamus, and cingulate gyrus; and a contralateral system—the lateral frontal cortex, particularly the premotor cortex, and parts of the basal ganglia. Boucsein goes on to propose that the ipsilateral component controls EDA when the stimulus is of an emotional or affective nature, and the contralateral component controls EDA during orienting, cognition, and locomotion. For more details of this model the reader is referred to Boucsein's comprehensive book.

Peripherally, we know that eccrine sweat glands (a special type of sweat gland) are intimately involved in EDA. Eccrine sweat glands are concentrated in the palms of the hands and soles of the feet. What makes them of particular interest to psychologists is that they respond primarily to "psychic" stimulation, whereas other sweat glands respond more to increases in temperature. The eccrine sweat glands are innervated by the sympathetic branch of the ANS, but the chemical transmitter at the post-ganglionic synapse is acetylcholine, not noradrenaline, as would be expected in the sympathetic nervous system (Shields, MacDowell, Fairchild, & Campbell, 1987). This is worth noting, because some investigators make the mistake of generalizing from EDA recording to all other psychophsyiological activity. Generalizing from one channel of data is always risky in psychophsyiology (see chapter 5), but particularly so when the single measure used is an exception to the rule.

The eccrine sweat glands, which can be thought of as tiny tubes with their openings at the surface of the skin, act as variable resistors wired in parallel. Figure 13.2 shows a simplified model. Depending upon the degree of sympathetic activation, sweat rises toward the surface of the skin in varying amounts and in varying numbers of sweat glands. The higher the sweat rises in a given gland, the lower the resistance in that variable resistor. In some cases, but certainly not all, sweat overflows onto the surface of the skin. This hydration of the skin with salty sweat increases SCL and SPL. Remember, conductance is the reciprocal of resistance. Years ago, it was thought that EDA was determined solely by the amount of sweat on the surface of the skin. We now know this is not so. Even in those cases where stimulation does not result in sweat at the surface of the skin, changes in EDA are often found because even a slight rise of the sweat in the glands will change the values of the variable resistors shown in figure 13.2. If we wished to quantify the EDA at a given moment, we would sum the values of all the active resistors that are wired in parallel. The sum of resistors in parallel equals the sum of their reciprocals, or conductance. This is one reason for using skin conductance rather than skin resistance when describing exosomatic EDA. A second reason, which will be discussed in the section on Analysis and Quantification, is that skin conductance, unlike skin resistance, does not have to be corrected for base level (see the discussion of the law of initial values in chapter 5). In addition to the hydration of the skin and

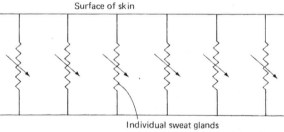

Individual sweat glands
conceptualized as variable resistors

Figure 13.2. A simplified model of sweat gland activity with the individual glands depicted as variable resistors wired in parallel.

the number of active sweat glands, other factors that may be involved in EDA include a membrane in the sweat duct wall that effects the reabsorption of sweat (Edelberg, 1972) and changes in pressure in the duct that effect the opening of the pores in the skin (Edelberg, 1993). And for skin potential, Christie and Venables (1971) demonstrated that SPL of extremely relaxed subjects is determined largely by the concentration of potassium at the surface of the skin.

## Skin Conductance

### Recording Procedure

*Electrodes*   Silver-silver chloride electrodes should be used to minimize polarization, which can affect the subject's conductance. The size of the electrodes will affect conductance; the size used should be stated. Standard commercial electrodes are a good size and attach conveniently with double-sided adhesive collars. The collars also help control the size of the skin area that comes in contact with the electrode jelly. The contact area, not the size of the electrode, effects the conductance values. Extremely small electrodes should be avoided, because the smaller the contact area the greater the current density (the amount of current flowing per unit of electrode area). Too high a current density will effect the recordings and could even stimulate underlying tissue.

The electrode jelly is the conductive medium between the electrodes and the skin. Commercial EKG or EEG electrode jellies can be used for SC recording, but if they contain near saturation concentrations of saline, such jellies will effect recordings over time. Instructions for making electrode jelly that will not effect recordings are given in Venables and Christie (1973, p. 80).

*Electrode Placement*   The electrodes are attached where the concentration of eccrine sweat glands is the highest—the palmar surface of the hands or fingers or the soles of the feet. Either bipolar or monopolar placements may be used. Figure 13.3(a) shows two typical bipolar placements. Figure 13.3(b) depicts a monopolar placement.

*Recording Equipment*   Older equipment for recording EDA impressed a direct current across two electrodes and indicated changes in skin resistance. Newer circuits, instead of imposing a constant current, impose a constant voltage, resulting in a direct readout of skin conductance. Either system can be used; in fact, they are both used in the same way. In the section on Common Problems, the conversion from resistance values (ohms) to conductance (microsiemens or the older term micromhos) is discussed. Considerable amplification is required to record what can be a

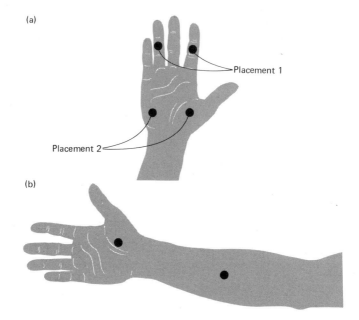

Figure 13.3. Typical bipolar and monopolar electrode placements. (a) Bipolar; (b) monopolar.

very weak signal. A reliable calibration signal (normally found in commercial skin conductance couplers) is also needed in order to quantify responses.

*Procedure* If bipolar electrodes are to be used, the chosen sites are simply washed with soap and water and the electrodes are attached. With monopolar placements, after both sites have been cleaned, the skin over the inactive site must be abraded. At the start of recording, the appropriate degree of amplification must be selected. One way to tell if there is sufficient gain is to have the subject take a deep breath. If no response is seen, the amplification should be increased. If, on the other hand, the record frequently goes off scale while the subject is relaxing, the gain is too high. After the desired amplification is set, the calibration signal should be recorded.

*Factors to Control When Recording EDA* The following subject variables have been found to effect EDA: age, sex, race, and stage of menstrual cycle. Environmental factors that effect EDA include temperature, humidity, time of day, day of week, and season. For a discussion of the specific effects of these variables, see Venables and Christie (1973) or Boucsein (1992).

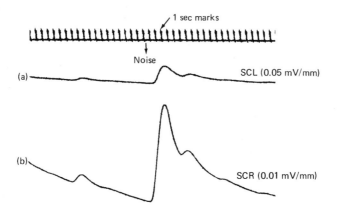

Figure 13.4. A simultaneous recording of SCL (a) and SCR (b) to a noise.

### Typical Recordings

Figure 13.4(a) shows the skin conductance level recorded on a low-amplification channel to a loud noise; figure 13.4(b) shows the same signal recorded on a second higher-amplification channel to obtain the skin conductance response. Figure 13.5 is a record of the spontaneous skin conductance activity of a subject considered to be a labile responder, that is, one who showed numerous responses for which there were no known stimuli.

### Common Problems

*Simultaneous Recording of Level and Response* If one is interested in simultaneously recording SC level and response, or SP level and response, then there is a problem. Basically, the problem is how to set one amplifier in order to amplify two signals, or two aspects of the same signal, when the signals or aspects vary greatly in magnitude. The amount of amplification needed in order to see the relatively small phasic responses will be much too great to observe the relatively large tonic level; the record will be driven off the scale by shifts in the tonic level. Before discussing methods for solving this problem, we should mention why one might

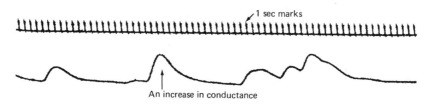

Figure 13.5. Spontaneous skin conductance activity.

want to record level and response simultaneously. One possibility is that the investigator might be interested in the two separate measures as a function of some stimulus situation. The more usual reason for simultaneous recording is an interest in phasic activity (the size of the discrete response), together with the realization that the size of the response is somewhat dependent on the tonic level prior to stimulation, particularly if skin resistance rather than conductance is recorded (see the discussion of the law of initial values in chapter 5).

One method of solving this recording problem is to split the signal coming from the subject. One signal is then fed into a high-amplification channel for SCR, and the other into a relatively low-amplification DC channel for SCL (see figure 13.4). But this method is expensive, because it requires two channels of equipment. An alternative method provides phasic and tonic information within one channel and is available on some commercial equipment. A bucking voltage or offsetting circuit is used. With the subject in the circuit, the experimenter turns a knob that is calibrated in units appropriate for measurement of tonic level, until the signal is zeroed. At this moment, the experimenter can read the size of the internal signal needed to oppose the subject's tonic level, the conductance level, or potential level. With amplification turned up, the experimenter can then observe the relatively small phasic responses.

*Converting from Resistance Readings to Conductance*  As previously stated, some older equipment provides output in terms of resistance (ohms) rather than conductance (micromhos). Note that the older unit of measurement for conductance "mhos" is "ohms" spelled backwards. The current unit of measurement for conductance is microsiemen or $\mu S$ (see table 13.1). The conversion itself is a simple matter, since resistance is the reciprocal of conductance. However, a warning is in order. Beware when converting the amplitude of a response from resistance to conductance. Do not subtract the poststimulus resistance from the prestimulus resistance and then convert the difference to conductance. Rather, convert the prestimulus resistance to conductance and convert the poststimulus resistance to conductance and then subtract the two conductances.

Figure 13.6 shows a typical response recorded on equipment that provides the output in resistance (ohms). The amplitude of the response in conductance units ($\mu S$) was obtained as follows:

$$\begin{aligned}
\text{Poststimulus level} &= 90{,}000 \text{ ohms} &&= 11\ \mu S \\
\text{Prestimulus level} &= 100{,}000 \text{ ohms} &&= 10\ \mu S \\
\text{Amplitude of response} & &&= 1\ \mu S
\end{aligned}$$

### Analysis and Quantification

*Amplitude*  Figure 13.7 shows typical skin conductance waveforms. Measurement of the amplitude of figure 13.7(a) is simple: conductance at the

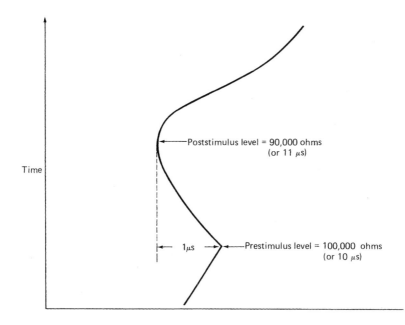

Figure 13.6. A typical response recorded on equipment that provides the output in resistance (ohms). The size of the response when converted to conductance is shown to be 1 μS.

peak minus conductance prior to the response. Difficulties arise, however, when a second response occurs before the first recovers, as in figure 13.7(b) or 13.7(d). One way of measuring the amplitude of the second wave in figure 13.7 (b) is shown in figure 13.7(c). Most psychophysiologists do not use this approach, however, preferring instead to measure the amplitude of each successive wave from its point of origin, as shown in figure 13.7(d).

When conductance change is used, it usually is not necessary to correct for base level conductance prior to the response. Table 13.2 shows why this is so. The skin resistance and skin conductance response of two hypothetical subjects are compared. Subject A's prestimulus level of resistance is very high compared to that of subject B. Therefore, it might be said that A's electrodermal system has much further to decrease than B's or that the size of B's responses should be inflated when compared with A's because of the differences in prestimulus level. Simplistically, it is easier for A to respond—show a decrease in resistance—than it is for B. In the example given, both subjects decreased 10,000 Ω. This was actually a much greater response for B, considering B's low prestimulus level; so, the size of the response must be "corrected." The lower half of table 13.2 shows the same data converted to conductance. Note that here the size of B's response is much greater than A's, as it should be.

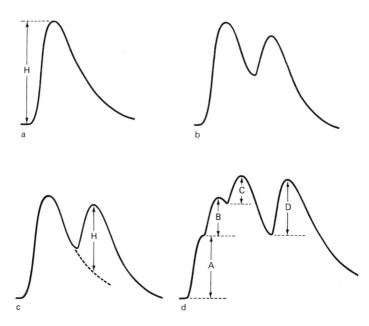

Figure 13.7. Criteria for measurement of skin conductance amplitude (H). Method d is preferred over method c for measurement of compound responses. Redrawn with permission from R. Edelberg, 1967, "Electrical properties of the skin." In C. C. Brown (Ed.), *Methods in psychophysiology*, Baltimore: Williams and Wilkins.

There is no need to correct the conductance data. Conductance data are usually relatively normally distributed, eliminating the need for a transformation.

One possible transformation that should be considered, however, has been described in detail by Lykken, Rose, Luther, and Maley (1966) and can be applied to all psychophysiological data. This technique enables us to express the amplitude of a response relative to a particular subject's minimum and maximum conditions of activation.

*Latency*   The latency of EDA refers to the time from stimulus to onset of the response. The latency of EDA is usually 1.0 to 3.0 s. It is difficult to measure accurately because SCR does not begin abruptly but instead starts gradually. This makes onset difficult to determine.

*Recovery Time*   The onset phase of an SCR—the time from the start of the response until it peaks—depends largely on the amplitude of the response and is, therefore, of little interest to most investigators. Edelberg (1972) and others suggest that the rate of recovery of an SCR is somewhat independent of amplitude, mediated by the central nervous system and of interest to psychologists. The specific measure of recovery time

Table 13.2. A Comparision of Skin Resistance and Skin Conductance Responses in Relationship to Prestimulus Levels

| | Resistance (ohms) | |
| --- | --- | --- |
| | Subject A | Subject B |
| Prestimulus | 100,000 | 20,000 |
| Poststimulus | 90,000 | 10,000 |
| Amplitude of response | 10,000 | 10,000 |
| | Conductance ($\mu$S) | |
| Prestimulus | 10 | 50 |
| Poststimulus | 11 | 100 |
| Amplitude of response | 1 | 50 |

used, rec t/2, is the time from the peak to the point at which the response has recovered to 50% amplitude. Numerous authors (e.g., Christie, 1976) relate the SCR recovery rate to the nature of the testing situation (e.g., threatening versus task-orienting) and to the nature of the subject (e.g, schizophrenics versus normals).

*Frequency*   Counting nonspecific SCRs is not as easy as it seems. First, one must set the criteria for a response; 0.01 $\mu$S is commonly used. Then one must rule out SCRs that occur within so many seconds of a known stimulus, such as a deep breath. We suggest discounting all ANS responses for approximately 20 s after such a disturbance (see Stern and Anschel, 1968).

## Skin Potential

### Recording Procedure

Endosomatic recording of EDA is performed with no excitation current. What is recorded is the skin potential over a site rich in eccrine sweat glands, with reference to an inactive site. The recording equipment must contain a stable, high-gain amplifier with a high-input impedance. Standard silver-silver chloride electrodes are used, as with SC recording. In SP recording, it is crucial to minimize electrode bias. The degree of bias, or difference in potential, between a pair of electrodes can be measured by immersing them in a saline solution and measuring the potential with the same high-input impedance recorder that will be used to measure

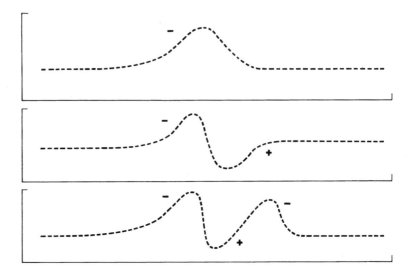

Figure 13.8. Three different waveforms commonly found in skin potential recording. Negativity is recorded upward by convention and amplitude is measured from the same prestimulus baseline.

skin potential. The bias potential should be less than 1 mV. The size of the electrodes is not critical. Monopolar placement must be used (figure 13.3), and the inactive site must be abraded. The basic recording procedure is similar to that used for the recording of SC.

*Typical Recordings*   Figure 13.8 shows three different waveforms commonly seen in SP recording. Note that negativity is recorded upward by convention; the top figure depicts a simple negative wave. The middle tracing shows a typical biphasic SP response. The lower figure shows a more unusual triphasic waveform.

## Common Problems

Electrode drift is the most common problem in recording skin potential. Since SP recording must be carried out with relatively high amplification, any slight potential between the electrodes will be recorded as a slow wave, indistinguishable from a slow change in skin potential level. As previously mentioned, electrode bias should be measured prior to recording. In addition, electrode bias should be checked after a recording session in order to be confident that the source of the record was the skin potential of the subject rather than electrode potential.

## Analysis and Quantification

*Amplitude* It is difficult to quantify the amplitude of SPRs. The conventional method of quantifying a biphasic response is to measure the negative response from the preresponse level to its peak and then measure the positive response from the same preresponse level to its peak (see figure 13.7). The difficulty is that the amplitude of the negative wave is attenuated, by some unknown amount, by the onset of the positive wave.

*Latency* Latency of the first wave of the SPR can be measured much like latency in SCR (as previously discussed). The values obtained should be similar.

### References

Boucsein, W. (1992). *Electrodermal activity*. New York: Plenum.

Christie, M. J. (1976). Electrodermal activity. In O. W. Hill (Ed.), *Modern trends in psychosomatic medicine. Vol. 3*. London: Butterworth.

Christie, M. J., & Venables, P. H. (1971). Characteristics of palmar skin potential and conductance in relaxed human subjects. *Psychophysiology, 8*, 523–532.

Darrow, C. W. (1933). The functional significance of the galvanic skin reflex and perspiration on the backs and palms of the hands. *Psychological Bulletin, 30*, 712.

Dawson, M. E., Schell, A. M. & Filion, L. (1990). The electrodermal system. In J. T. Cacioppo and L. G. Tassinary (Eds.), *Principles of psychophysiology* (pp. 295–324). Cambridge: Cambridge University Press.

Edelberg, R. (1967). Electrical properties of the skin. In C. C. Brown (Ed.), *Methods in psychophysiology* (pp. 1–53). Baltimore: Williams & Wilkins.

Edelberg, R. (1972). The electrodermal system. In N. S. Greenfield & R. A. Sternbach (Eds.), *Handbook of psychophysiology* (pp. 367–418). New York: Holt, Rinehart & Winston.

Edelberg, R. (1973). Mechanisms of electrodermal adaptations for locomotion, manipulation, or defense. In E. Stellar and J. M. Sprague (Eds.), *Progress in physiological psychology Vol. 5* (pp. 155–209). New York: Academic Press.

Edelberg, R. (1993). Electrodermal mechanisms: A critique of the two-effector hypothesis and a proposed replacement. In J. C. Roy, W. Boucsein, D. C. Fowles, & J. H. Gruzelier (Eds.), *Progress in electrodermal research* (pp. 7–30). New York: Plenum.

Jung, C. G. (1907). On psychophysical relations of the associative experiment. *Journal of Abnormal Psychology, 7*, 247–255.

Lykken, D. T., Rose, R., Luther, B., & Maley, M. (1966). Correcting pychophysiological measures for individual differences in range. *Psychological Bulletin, 66*, 481–484.

Lykken, D. T., & Venables, P. H. (1971). Direct measurement of skin conductance: A proposal for standardization. *Psychophysiology, 8*, 656–672.

Neumann, E., & Blanton, R. (1970). The early history of electrodermal research. *Psychophysiology, 6,* 453–475.

Peterson, F. (1907). The galvanometer as a measure of emotions. *British Medical Journal, 2,* 804–806.

Shields, S. A., MacDowell, K. A., Fairchild, S. B., & Campbell, M. L. (1987). Is mediation of sweating cholernergic, adrenergic, or both? A comment on the literature. *Psychophysiology, 24,* 312–319.

Siddle, D. A. T. (1991). Orienting, habituation, and resource allocation: An associative analysis. *Psychophysiology, 28,* 245–259.

Stern, R. M., & Anschel, C. (1968). Deep inspirations as stimuli for responses of the autonomic nervous system. *Psychophysiology, 5,* 132–141.

Venables, P. H., & Christie, M. H. (1973). Mechanisms, instrumentation, recording techniques, and quantification of responses. In W. F. Prokasy and D. C. Raskin (Eds.), *Electrodermal activity in psychological research* (pp. 2–124). New York: Academic Press.

# 14

## Signal Processing

You have designed a cognitive intervention intended to increase attentional abilities in young children. You would like to use a psychophysiological method to determine if there are any effects of your intervention on attentional control. Before you begin a study, you will need to choose the psychophysiological variable(s) that will permit you to answer your question. You base this decision on the conceptualization of your research question and on what is known about the impact of the relevant psychological variable (e.g., attention) on the measured physiological variable(s). In this case, because your question concerns possible changes in attentional ability, you will want to choose a dependent variable that reflects changes in attentional processes.

The next important issue is to decide, for each measured physiological variable, whether you are interested in recording basal (tonic) activity or event-related (phasic) activity (see chapter 4). What is considered to be the basal or tonic level of activity in a physiological system is typically determined by your question and by the physiological system of interest. In general, you can derive tonic activity from the ongoing level of activity in the system when the organism is at rest. The length of time needed to assess tonic level appropriately will differ across physiological systems, but in many cases it will be on the order of several minutes. Time periods shorter than this can be unstable measures of tonic activity because of the occurrence of phasic events that can drastically alter the mean value of physiological function during the period. On the other hand, time periods longer than this are often difficult to obtain because subjects do not like to sit still for more than a few minutes, and very long time periods (i.e., hours) may be altered by circadian effects. Phasic responses typically are measured over time periods that capture the full response from basal level until the physiological parameter returns to it's basal level. The speed with which a physiological system responds and activity returns

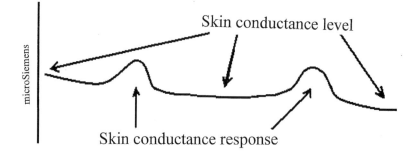

Figure 14.1. Sample analog skin conductance signal. Both basal skin conductance levels and two skin conductance responses are depicted (units are microSiemens).

to baseline differs from system to system. As we mentioned in chapter 13, eccrine sweat gland activity measured as skin conductance is an example of a system from which one can record both tonic and phasic activity. Basal skin conductance, also referred to as skin conductance level, changes relatively slowly (i.e., several seconds to minutes; see figure 14.1). In addition, skin conductance can also show short-term changes known as skin conductance responses, which are superimposed on this background skin conductance level. These responses typically last several seconds and are distinct from the background level of activity (figure 14.1). Skin conductance responses may be nonspecific, (meaning that we do not know of any event leading to their occurrence) or responses can be event-related (meaning that the skin conductance response appears to have occurred as a result of an experimenter-controlled external event such as a stimulus display, or an unplanned or subject-controlled event such as a sneeze).

Your decision about whether to record physiological level or response (or both) will influence your recording parameters. First, you'll need to determine the length of the time period that you wish to record. Note that if you want to measure tonic activity then the recording period is likely to be long relative to what is required to record a response. For example, skin conductance or heart rate level is often determined over one to several minutes, whereas a phasic skin conductance or heart rate response is determined over one to several seconds. The time period length should be based on what is known about the tonic levels and phasic responsiveness of the physiological system of interest. Second, you will need to decide on a *sampling rate* at which you want to record the signal. Sampling rate, measured as samples per second, refers to the rate at which your original (analog) physiological signal is converted to a digital form, or set of numbers, by a computer (figure 14.2). The analog signal is a waveform that is continuous across time. When the computer

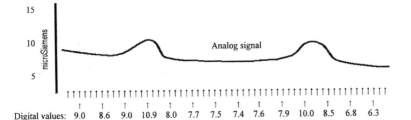

Figure 14.2. Sample analog skin conductance signal and some digital values illustrating sampling. A sample (a conversion from the analog signal to a digital value) is taken at each vertical arrow over time. Every fourth digital value is shown below the analog signal. Digital values are shown in microSiemen units.

samples the signal it assigns a numerical (digital) value based on the current value of the analog signal. In order to reproduce the original signal accurately in digital form, it is important to sample frequently enough so that the signal is reproduced faithfully. In figure 14.3, the lower panel depicts a digital reconstruction of the analog signal depicted in the upper panel. Notice that if you sample too slowly, the recreated, digitized signal will not look like the original, analog signal. Also note that although there are lines drawn between the dots, that the only

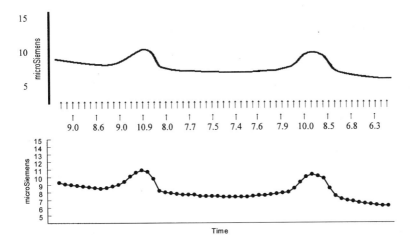

Figure 14.3. Sample analog skin conductance signal (upper panel) and the recreated digital signal (lower panel). Each digital sample is represented by a solid circle in the lower panel and the samples are connected by a line. Note that when the signal level changes rapidly, the sampling rate shown is less able to recreate faithfully the original analog signal than when the signal changes slowly.

information one has in a digitized signal are the data points represented by the dots (which are numbers). Indeed, a digitized signal is also known as a discrete-time signal because we only know the values of the signal at discrete time points, and not at the points in between. Thus, the illustration of a signal using "connect-the-dots" is a depiction only; we cannot know for sure what the values of the analog signal are between the sampled points. In order to reproduce all of the elements of interest from the analog signal in the digitized waveform, one needs to determine the highest frequency component of interest in the signal. As we mentioned in chapter 3, it is necessary to sample at least twice the highest frequency of interest in order to reproduce the signal; in general, it is a good idea to sample even faster than that (e.g., four to eight times the highest frequency of interest; Cacioppo, Tassinary & Fridlund, 1990). This rule requiring a sampling rate of at least twice the highest frequency component in the signal is referred to as the *Nyquist relation*. When sampling is too slow, a digital form of the physiological signal will be produced that does not accurately represent the original signal which is a problem known as *aliasing* (figure 14.4). It may seem surprising, but recording period length and sampling rate are related issues because the memory capacity limitations of a computer used for collecting physiological data results in a trade-off between these two experimental parameters. The longer one's recording time, the more memory is required in order to store the physiological data. Likewise, the faster the sampling rate, the more numbers must be stored per unit of time and the greater the memory requirements for the computer storing the data.

One final decision that should be made prior to data collection is whether you will use a filter when collecting the data. Filters remove, or filter out, unwanted frequencies of activity from your physiological signals. One of the most important sources of unwanted variation that can be removed using a filter is 60 Hz noise. Such noise arises from electrical devices, computer screens, and a variety of other sources. Fluorescent lighting, a 120 Hz noise source, is particularly problematic in the psychophysiology lab. In general, it is better to shield the source of the noise from the subject or to shield the subject from the noise. However, in some circumstances, the environment may not be easily alterable. In this case, unwanted noise can be removed by filtering it out of the recorded signal. In addition to removing unwanted noise, filters can remove other unnecessary frequencies from the data. For example, when recording an EEG, one may want to examine a particular frequency of activity such as alpha activity in the EEG, but alpha activity may not be apparent to the unaided eye. However, a filter could be applied to remove frequencies above and below the alpha band, permitting a relatively clear view of predominantly alpha activity. Analog filters can be applied either online (during data collection), or digital filters can be applied using a computer either online or offline (after the data

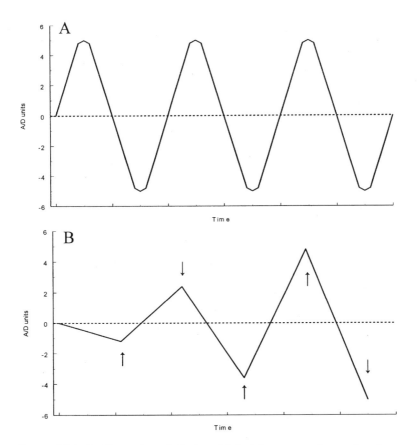

Figure 14.4. An illustration of aliasing: (a) depicts an exemplar analog physiological signal; (b) depicts a digital recreation of the original signal where a
sample was recorded at each vertical arrow. Note that the sampling rate was
too slow to recreate faithfully the original signal, a problem known as aliasing.

collection). Filters can be achieved either using electronic circuitry (i.e.,
a hardware filter) or using mathematical procedures such as FFT (discussed later in this chapter) which are based in software. A hardware
filter is typically applied when the data are collected, however, a software
filter can be applied to the data as they are collected or afterward. If
one is unsure of the effect of a chosen filter on the data, it is most
conservative to record the data unfiltered, and then to apply the filter
after data collection and check what effect the filter has on the data.
Investigators should also be cautious that filters do not remove desired
elements of a physiological signal; they should also be aware that filters
are not perfect: a 60 Hz filter removes some frequencies of activity around
60 Hz along with the 60 Hz activity.

In the days before computers were a ubiquitous part of the psycho-physiology laboratory, physiological signals were typically recorded with a polygraph and scored from a paper record by hand. Today, computers and relatively inexpensive recording equipment, and computer programs for collecting and reducing physiological signals make it possible for most labs to collect data directly into a computer and reduce the data offline after the experiment is over. After collecting your physiological data, the next step is to *reduce* it. Reducing physiological data refers to the process by which the large sets of numbers recorded by the computer are reduced to a smaller set of numbers that represent the events of interest during the experiment. For instance, although you may have sampled a plethys-mographic signal at 250 samples/s, you may ultimately decide that the numbers you want to use in a statistical analysis are the mean values of the plethysmographic signal for each 1-min period in the data set. Thus, you will reduce the large data set of numbers (i.e., the digitized signal representing the plethysmographic signal at 250 samples/s) to a set of numbers representing the mean value of the signal once per minute. Indeed, signal averaging is a very common method for reducing noise in data (for an example, see chapter 7 on event-related potentials). These averaged values then are submitted to statistical analyses and/or are plotted in graphical form in order to see changes as a result of your experimental manipulation or to see differences across different individ-uals. Next we will consider some of the ways in which you can assess your reduced physiological data.

## Assessing Basal Activity

Assessing basal or tonic activity is typically accomplished by computing mean values over a predefined period within the experiment. Mean values typically provide a reasonably representative view of the overall level of activity of the signal of interest. For some physiological signals, or under some circumstances, one may choose another measure of central ten-dency such as the median. The median is less sensitive than the mean to outliers in a data set. Thus, for data sets containing a sufficient number of outliers that the mean and median differ considerably, one may get a better estimate of the general level of activity using the median rather than the mean. In addition, one should be sensitive to whether an outlier (or group of outliers) could be a "real" physiological phenomenon (e.g., a severe bradycardia in an infant) or a result of movement-related or other artifact-related perturbation of the digitizing process. One may wish even to remove a "real" event, for instance a precipitous bradycardia, for purposes of creating a meaningful representation of the average level of activity without the influence of a single punctate event. One final issue concerns the choice of measure both for representing the status of the physiological system and for performing statistical analyses. Each physiological system will require a different solution for choosing a unit of measurement and deciding whether there is a need to transform the measurements for analysis purposes. When possible, it is suggested that units of measurement be chosen on the basis of the characteristics of the physiological system of interest (Levey, 1980). For an example, see the rationale given in chapter 12 for choosing heart period instead of heart rate as the cardiac metric. For more specific recommendations on the choice of units of measurement for physiological variables, the reader is urged to consult the relevant chapters in this volume. The reader should also consult the literature for relevant information on the following general measurement issues (Levey, 1980) and discussions on measurement of skin conductance (Boucsein, 1993; Fowles et al., 1981; Lykken & Venables, 1971), cardiac function (Berntson, Cacioppo & Quigley, 1995), electromyography (Cacioppo, Tassinary & Fridlund, 1990), ocular responses (Stern & Dunham, 1990), respiratory responses (Lorig & Schwartz, 1990), and sexual responses (Geer & Head, 1990).

## Assessing Change

Decisions about how to assess changes in physiology are somewhat more difficult than those for assessing tonic levels of activity. As we have mentioned previously, this is partly due to the fact that, in some cases, the amplitude of a response may be in part dependent on the baseline level of activity. We will discuss several of the methods used for assessing change and indicate some of the advantages and disadvantages associated with each measure.

### Change Scores

Change scores are computed by taking a measure during a phasic response (either the mean or the peak) and subtracting a measure of baseline activity. Thus, change scores reflect the change from the baseline to the response. The use of change scores has been debated in the psychological literature, with no firm consensus emerging for different physiological measures. This is because several issues influence whether or not a change score is a reliable measure of change in a physiological system over time. One issue concerns whether the baseline and task levels of activity are independent of one another. This issue is related to the *law of initial values* (LIV) (see chapter 5). The LIV states that the initial state of a system will limit the degree to which the system can change it's state. More specifically, the LIV states that the higher the basal level of function in a given physiological system, the more the system can decrease its function or the less the system can increase its function. The reverse is true when the basal level is low. There are situations in which physiological limits do impose a constraint on the amount of change (see Berntson, Uchino & Cacioppo, 1994). For example, there are physiological and metabolic limits on the rate with which the heart can beat and under normal physiological conditions there is a maximal rate. However, it is also clear that the LIV does not *always* occur. That is why we prefer to call it a "principle"; see also Myrtek and Foerster (1986). It is important to keep in mind that when physiological functions are near a "ceiling" or "floor" (i.e., near their physical limits), that responses can be constrained by the system. At least with regard to cardiovascular measures, within many typical laboratory reactivity paradigms the correlation between the baseline and the change score appears to be small, suggesting that the LIV is not consistently problematic (Llabre et al., 1991; Seraganian et al., 1985). However, the most conservative approach is probably to assess whether the baseline and task levels are correlated, and if so, decide if it is important to remove the effect of the baseline using one of the techniques discussed here.

The second issue concerns the issue of test-retest reliability of change scores. Test-retest reliability refers to the idea that a change score measured in a person in response to a task on one occasion should be similar to the change score measured in that same person in response to the same task on another occasion. If a measure is unreliable, it means that we cannot be sure that one would see a similar change score within a person if the study was completed again. In cardiovascular reactivity studies, where one typically measures changes in cardiovascular function as a result of a task, challenge or stressor, the reliability of change scores has been assessed. Cardiovascular measures such as heart rate and systolic blood pressure have been shown to have relatively good reliability, whereas diastolic blood pressure has poorer reliability (Llabre et al., 1991; Seraganian et al., 1985). For a discussion of reliability for several psychophysiological measures, see Tomarken (1995).

### Residualized Change Scores and Covariance Analyses

Residualized change scores are scores derived by computing a regression equation that reveals the relationship between the phasic or task level and the baseline level. Task level is regressed onto baseline level; then the difference between the expected value depicted by the regression line and the observed value becomes the new residualized change score (see figure 14.5). These change scores are sometimes used when there is a relationship between the task and baseline levels and the investigator wishes to remove the effect of the baseline. Note that unlike change scores (i.e., task − baseline), the residualized change score is dependent on the sample from which it is drawn. All data in the sample will be used to construct the re-

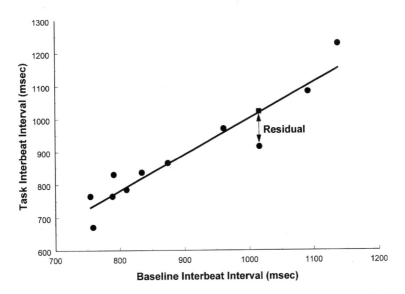

Figure 14.5. Derivation of a residual change score. As an example, task-level heart rates were regressed onto baseline-level heart rates. The residual is the difference (in bpm) between the observed value (solid circles) and the expected value for the baseline level (dark square). The expected value falls on the regression line that best fits the task and baseline level data. The residual represents the heart rate change that occurs independent of the baseline.

gression equation from which the residuals are derived; therefore, differences across samples will result in somewhat different regression equations, and thus residual scores will vary from sample to sample. In this regard, change scores are easier to interpret than residualized change scores, because they are comparable across studies. A technique that is conceptually similar to the use of residualized changes scores is analysis of covariance (ANCOVA). Using ANCOVA, one can use the baseline level as a covariate of the task level and thus statistically "remove" the effects of the baseline from the task level. Comparisons of change scores and residualized change scores in cardiovascular reactivity research suggest that they are usually similar in reliability; thus, the simple change score is sometimes recommended because of its ease of interpretation and calculation (Kamarck et al., 1992; Llabre et al., 1991; Manuck et al., 1989). Again, however, the best strategy is to assess the relationship between the baseline and task levels so that one can make an educated decision about whether or not to remove the effects of the baseline.

### Percent Change Scores

Another type of change score that is used is the percent change score. It is calculated by dividing the difference between the task and the baseline by the baseline (i.e., [task level − baseline level]/baseline level). Thus, the change in physiological activity is now represented as a function of the original baseline level. There are some caveats that should be considered when using percent change scores. First, percent change scores typically are not normally distributed, making them difficult to use in parametric statistical tests unless they are first transformed. Furthermore, the necessity of a transformation for statistical purposes after already making the percentage transformation means that the data have now been transformed twice and thus have become difficult to understand in the sense of "real world" interpretability. Finally, little work has been done assessing the reliability of percent change scores. Because of the difficulty of interpreting transformed percent change scores and a lack of information on their reliability, percent change scores are not usually recommended unless the investigator can provide evidence of reliability.

## Assessing Global Aspects of Physiological Signals

Recent advances in signal processing capabilities with computers allow the psychophysiologist to assess easily more global aspects of a physiological signal. These techniques can provide an overall look at the variation in the signal over time, the frequency of that variation, and whether the variation forms an overall pattern that is not visible to the naked eye. Analytical tools that permit examination of a signal over time are called *time domain techniques*. Tools that permit the investigator to examine the frequency characteristics of a signal are called *frequency domain techniques*. Time domain techniques tend to be useful for showing what a signal looks like over time. However, low-frequency patterns in a signal, particularly in a signal recorded over a very long time period, can be difficult to envision using time domain techniques. Instead, frequency domain techniques often provide a more useful way of characterizing a physiological signal because they serve to unearth patterns in the data that are not visible to the eye. The interested reader is urged to consult sources that can give a more detailed explanation of the various techniques detailed here; useful sources of additional information are suggested in each section. For an accessible overview of digital signal processing, the reader is urged to consult Lyons (1997).

### Fourier Analysis or Fast Fourier Transforms

Biological signals are typically composed of complex-looking waveforms. Sometimes, we may want to decompose those waveforms into their component frequencies because we believe that there is biological and/or psychological "meaning" associated with a particular frequency of activity. For instance, there is an oscillation in heart period that is coincident with the respiratory frequency (approximately 0.12–0.4 Hz in adult humans). This oscillation in heart period (or heart rate) is due to central nervous system respiratory oscillators and feedback from the lungs, and under some circumstances this oscillation will have a visible impact on the heart period matching the frequency of respiration (see figure 12.5). The oscillation appears to be associated with central parasympathetic outflow to the heart; thus it is a frequency of particular interest for some psychophysiologists (see chapter 12 for more information).

Fast Fourier Transform (FFT) is a frequency domain procedure by which physiological signals comprised of waveforms with different frequencies and different amplitudes are decomposed so that one can observe the underlying frequencies that make up the signal. The FFT assumes that the underlying waveforms are sine waves; although this is not necessarily a correct assumption for biological signals, it can still serve as a reasonable approximation to reality. The FFT process is analogous to taking sine waves of many different frequencies and seeing how each of the sine waves fits the signal of interest. Mathematically, the FFT steps through a series of sine waves of successively greater frequencies, checking a template of each frequency against the signal and quantifying how much of the signal matches each of the frequency templates. The FFT results in a graphical depiction called the power spectrum or spectral density plot that illustrates how a given signal sampled over time is decomposed into it's component sine waves which differ in frequency and amplitude. The spectral density plot is useful because it summarizes how much activity in the original signal arose from each frequency of sine wave that was fitted to the signal. Figures 14.6 and 14.7 depict the "template-matching" that is performed by an FFT. Notice that each of the templates matches some part of the original signal, but that some frequencies contribute more to the original signal than others. The spectral density plot that results shows which frequency templates were most prominent in the signal (i.e., greater power), and those which were a small component of the signal (i.e., less power). Figure 14.8 shows time domain and frequency domain depictions of two single frequency sine waves and a signal made up of the two individual sine waves. Figure 14.8 (a) and 14.8 (b) each show a sine wave of one frequency and amplitude. The left panels of the figure show the sine waves in the time domain and the right panels show the decomposed sine wave in the frequency domain. Figure 14.8 (c) depicts the combination of the sine waves shown in figure 14.8 (a) and 14.8 (b) and illustrates how the decomposition of the signal in the frequency domain reveals both frequency components (one at $f_0$ and the other at $2 f_0$). Figure 14.9 illustrates two different frequency domain depictions, one showing amplitude and the other showing power (or spectral density) of the data shown in the right side of figure 14.8 (c). Figure 14.9 shows that the signal is made up of two different frequencies and that the amplitudes and spectral power of the two frequency components differ. Indeed, power is simply the (amplitude)$^2$.

Biological signals are not made up simply of sine waves. FFT can still be used, however, as long as the investigator is aware that the interpretation of the power spectra for biological signals is less straightforward than the interpretation of power spectra produced for pure sine waves. Some real physiological signals (heart period and respiration) are depicted in figure 14.10 and demonstrate that the resulting power spectra will be more complex (e.g., has more than one peak) for more complex physiological signals. Thus, respiration, which is relatively sinusoidal for a physiological signal, gives a relatively clean, single-peaked power spectrum. However, heart period, which is composed of multiple frequency components, gives a more complex, multipeaked power spectrum. There are other computational issues that must be addressed when using FFT, such as the need to window the signals to remove the abrupt frequency shifts that can occur at the beginning and end of a recording period, which the investigator should understand when performing FFT analyses. For a discussion of the issues related to using time domain and frequency domain analyses such as FFT with psychophysiological signals, see Por-

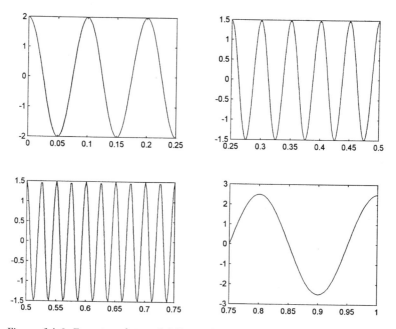

Figure 14.6. Four templates of different frequencies that were used to construct the signal shown in the top panel of Fig. 14.7.

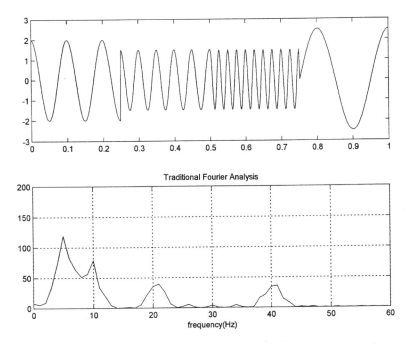

Figure 14.7. The top panel illustrates a curve constructed from the templates shown in figure 14.6. The bottom panel illustrates a spectral analysis (FFT) of the signal in the upper panel with four characteristic frequencies emerging as peaks.

ges & Bohrer (1990) for a very thorough treatment of the methodological issues and caveats for interpretation. For illustrations of the use of FFTs to analyze EGG signals, see chapter 11 and Stern, Koch, and Vasey (1990). The reader desiring additional information about FFTs should consult Lyons (1997, chapter 4).

### Coherence Analysis

At times researchers are interested in the question of how two separate physiological signals might be related. The two panels of figure 14.10 depict data from respiration and the heart. Although the graphs suggest that the signals are similar, there are computational methods which can help you to determine how similar they are. One method is that of coherence (see Porges & Bohrer, 1990, for a description of the method). An easy way to understand coherence is to see it as a correlation procedure for relating two signals. In addition, the correlation is squared and thus coherence values range from 0 to 1.00. The upper panel of figure 14.11 shows the same data depicted in figure 14.10. However, the lower panel of figure 14.11 now shows a coherence plot of the two signals in the upper panel. To provide a better understanding of coherence, let us take another example: brain activity, namely EEG. In this case we want to know if two signals coming from two parts of the brain are similar. You might first ask if the two signals are of the same frequency. The measure of coherence gives you the answer to this question by determining the frequency components that make up each signal (like an FFT analysis) and then examining the correlation between the two signals at each frequency. Thus, two signals can be alike at one frequency but not necessarily at another. You can also have a situation in which the signal recorded over one part of the brain is similar to that over another part except that the signals do not occur synchronously—instead one signal is delayed behind the other one. A coherence analysis

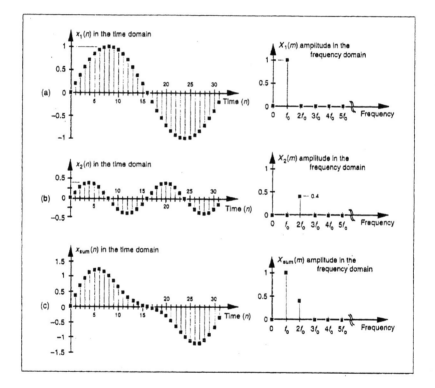

Figure 14.8. Time and frequency domain depictions of sine waves. The left panels illustrate sine waves in the time domain and the frequency domain characterizations of those waves are shown in the right panels. (a) A sine wave with an amplitude of 1 and a frequency of $f_0$. (b) A sine wave with an amplitude of 0.4 and a frequency of $2f_0$. (c) The sum of the two sine waves shown in (a) and (b) and how both frequencies and amplitudes are revealed by the frequency domain depiction on the right. Reprinted with permission from R. G. Lyons, 1997, *Understanding digital signal processing*, Reading, MA: Addison-Wesley.

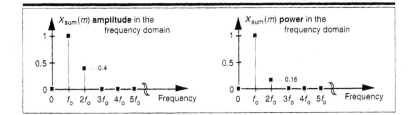

Figure 14.9. Two frequency domain depictions of sine waves. These frequency domain illustrations are based on the sine waves shown in Figure 14.8. The left panel is identical to the depiction in the right side of Figure 14.8 (c) and illustrates the amplitude and frequency components of the sum of two sine waves. The right panel shows a different frequency domain depiction where amplitude has been squared to produce power. This depiction shows the result of a FFT analysis. Reprinted with permission from R. G. Lyons, 1997, *Understanding digital signal processing*, Reading, MA: Addison-Wesley.

can detect this delay or lag between two signals (called the phase angle). Using this analysis we could determine that EEG over one brain region is delayed by some defined period from that over another region. An example of the use of coherence analysis of the EEG during a movement task can be found in Ford, Goethe, and Dekker (1986).

### Wavelet Analysis

Wavelet analysis can be viewed as being similar to Fourier analysis in that they are both means of transforming data unfolding over time into a series of frequency components. However, wavelet analysis can be used to assess the frequency components of data that are not amenable to Fourier analysis, which is problematic for viewing short-term changes in a physiological signal. Indeed, FFT requires a signal to be relatively stable or stationary over the time period from which frequency components are derived.

Figure 14.12 shows the output of a wavelet analysis (bottom plot) for a signal (top plot) that changes in frequency during the time period. Notice how the changes in the signal are reflected immediately in the wavelet analysis. The basic idea is that rather than examining a signal in terms of sine waves of varying frequencies (as in FFT), various time segments of the signal are instead viewed as shifted and scaled versions of a particular mathematical function, namely, the wavelet. Such a procedure is useful for examining in detail an aspect of the physiological signal that is different from that preceding and following it. For example, if you were to look at the optical illusion that consists either of two faces or a vase depending on your perception, wavelet analysis would allow you to examine the EEG both before and after the optical illusion switched from one perception to the other. Figure 14.13 shows such an analysis of the change in EEG with the "flipping" of a Necker cube illusion from one perspective to the other. For a recent discussion of the use of wavelet analysis see Samar, Bopardikar, Rao, and Swartz (1999).

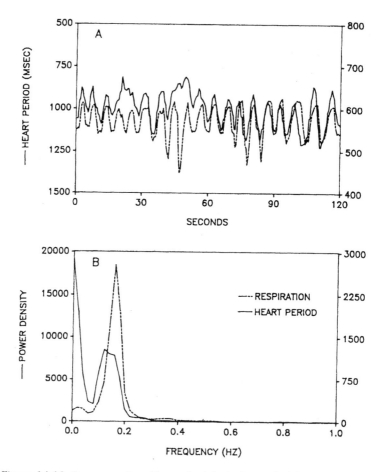

Figure 14.10. Power spectra of two physiological signals. (a) Two physiological signals, respiration and heart period, over a 2-min period. (b) The power density spectra for the two physiological signals shown in (a). Note the close concordance between the prominent peak in the respiratory spectrum and the higher frequency peak in the heart period spectrum. These peaks co-occur with the predominant respiratory frequency. Reprinted with permission from S. W. Porges and R. E. Bohrer, 1990, "The analysis of periodic processes in psychophysiological research." In J. T. Cacioppo and L. G. Tassinary (Eds.); *Principles of psychophysiology: Physical, social and inferential elements*, New York: Cambridge University Press.

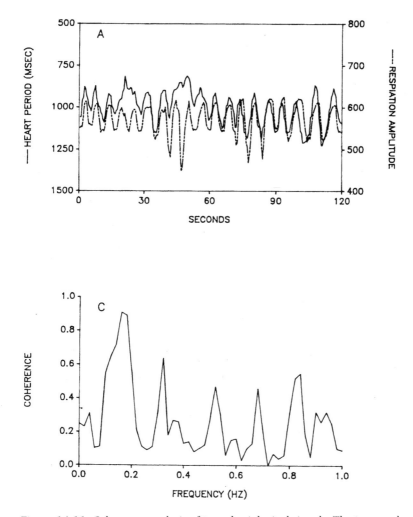

Figure 14.11. Coherence analysis of two physiological signals. The top panel shows the respiration and heart period data from Figure 14.10. The bottom panel depicts the coherence analysis between the respiration and heart period. Note that coherence is high (i.e., the correlation is strong) over some portions of the epoch, but weaker over other portions. Reprinted with permission from S. W. Porges and R. E. Bohrer, 1990, "The analysis of periodic processes in psychophysiological research." In J. T. Cacioppo and L. G. Tassinary (Eds.), *Principles of psychophysiology: Physical, social, and inferential elements*, New York: Cambridge University Press.

## Nonlinear Dynamical Systems (Chaos) Analysis

In contrast to the traditional signal processing procedures that decompose a signal like the EEG into its component frequencies and thus reflect a limited amount of information (one dimensional), the dynamical systems view suggests that a time series reflects the effects of all other variables participating in the dynamics of the system. The theoretical basis for this view derives from a variety of mathematical theorems (e.g., Whitney embedding theorem). Given that complex dynamic systems (such as the human nervous system) have an enormous number of interrelated dependent variables which are impossible to measure directly, the theorems suggest that if we can measure any single variable with sufficient accuracy, sufficiently often, and for sufficiently long periods of time, then it is possible to make quantitatively meaningful inferences about the dynamic structure of the entire system from the behavior of that single variable. From this perspective we have a theoretical foundation to explain why the nonlinear dynamic or *chaotic* approach may offer a characterization of behavior that is richer than that obtained by classical measures. One important nonlinear, dynamical measure of interest is that of dimensionality, referred to as *d*. A periodic oscillation (e.g., a sine wave) would have a dimension of 1. A quasi-periodic oscillation (e.g., two disproportionate frequencies) would result in a dimension of 2. Truly random noise would have a dimension approaching infinity. Many studies have used dimensionality as a measure of neural processing. Lutzenberger, Preissl, and Pulvermuller (1995) suggest that the dimensionality measure represents a relative measure of the number of neural ensembles recruited

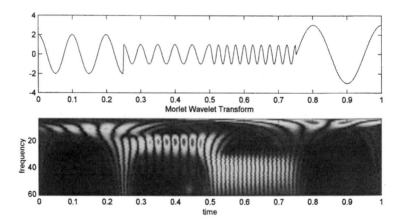

Figure 14.12. Output of a wavelet analysis (bottom plot) for a signal (top plot) that changes in frequency quickly during the time period. Notice how the changes in the signal are reflected immediately in the wavelet analysis.

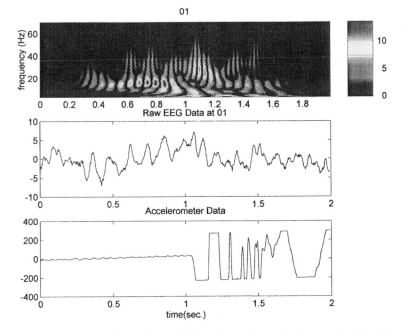

Figure 14.13. Wavelet analysis of EEG as the Necker cube illusion "switched." The top plot represents the output of the wavelet analysis in terms of time and frequency. The middle plot is EEG data recorded at the left occipital site of the scalp. The participant moved her finger slightly when the Necker cube "switched"; this was measured with an accelerometer, as shown in the bottom panel.

during a specific cognitive task. Applying this thinking on a global brain level, one might, for example, expect to see creativity to be associated with greater dimensionality. In terms of cardiovascular processes, given that the healthy heart shows greater variability than the abnormal one, one important question is whether regularity or the lack of nonlinear processing might be associated with the lack of health. An interesting theoretical application of the nonlinear approach is that of psychopathology (Globus & Arpaia, 1994). For an introduction to nonlinear dynamics especially in relation to physiology, see Elbert et al. (1994); Pritchard & Duke (1995); and Theiler (1990).

*References*

Berntson, G. G., Cacioppo, J. T., & Quigley, K. S. (1995). The metrics of cardiac chronotropism: Biometric perspectives. *Psychophysiology, 32,* 162–171.

Berntson, G. G., Uchino, B. N., & Cacioppo, J. T. (1994). Origins of baseline variance and the Law of Initial Values. *Psychophysiology, 31,* 204–210.

Boucsein, W. (1993). Methodological issues in electrodermal measurement. In J.-C. Roy, W. Boucsein, Fowles, D. C. & J. H. Gruzelier (Eds.), *Progress in electrodermal research* (pp. 31–41). New York: Plenum.

Cacioppo, J. T., Tassinary, L. G., & Fridlund, A. J. (1990). The skeletomotor system. In J. T. Cacioppo & L. G. Tassinary (Eds.), *Principles of psychophysiology: Physical, social, and inferential elements* (pp. 325–384). New York: Cambridge University Press.

Elbert, T., Ray, W., Kowalik, Z., Skinner, S., Graf, K., & Birbaumer, N. (1994). Chaos and Physiology. *Physiological Reviews, 74,* 1–47.

Ford, M. R., Goethe, J. W., & Dekker, D. K. (1986). EEG coherence and power changes during a continuous movement task. *International Journal of Psychophysiology, 4,* 99–110.

Fowles, D. C., Christie, M. J., Edelberg, R., Grings, W. W., Lykken, D. T., & Venables, P. H. (1981). Publication recommendations for electrodermal measurements. *Psychophysiology, 18,* 232–239.

Geer, J. H., & Head, S. (1990). The sexual response system. In J. T. Cacioppo & L. G. Tassinary (Eds.), *Principles of psychophysiology: Physical, social, and inferential elements* (pp. 599–630). New York: Cambridge University Press.

Globus, G., & Arpaia, J. (1994) Psychiatry and the new dynamics. *Biological Psychiatry, 35,* 352–364.

Kamarck, T. W., Jennings, J. R., Debski, T. T., Glickman-Weiss, E., Johnson, P. S., Eddy, M. J., & Manuck, S. B. (1992). Reliable measures of behaviorally-evoked cardiovascular reactivity from a PC-based test battery: Results from student and community samples. *Psychophysiology, 29,* 17–28.

Levey, A. B. (1980). Measurement units in psychophysiology. In I. Martin & P. H. Venables (Eds.), *Techniques in psychophysiology* (pp. 597–628). New York: Wiley.

Llabre, M. M., Spitzer, S. B., Saab, P. G., Ironson, G. H., & Schneiderman, N. (1991). The reliability and specificity of delta versus residualized change as measures of cardiovascular reactivity to behavioral challenges. *Psychophysiology, 28,* 701–711.

Lorig, T. S., & Schwartz, G. E. (1990). The pulmonary system. In J. T. Cacioppo & L. G. Tassinary (Eds.), *Principles of psychophysiology: Physical, social, and inferential elements* (pp. 580–598). New York: Cambridge University Press.

Lutzenberger, W., Preissl, H., & Pulvermuller, F. (1995). Fractal dimension electroencephalographic time series and underlying brain process. *Biological Cybernetics, 73,* 477–482.

Lykken, D. & Venables, P. H. (1971). Direct measurement of skin conductance: A proposal for standardization. *Psychophysiology, 14,* 329–331.

Lyons, R. G. (1997). *Understanding digital signal processing.* Reading, MA: Addison-Wesley.

Manuck, S. B., Kasprowicz, A. L., Monroe, S. M., Larkin, K. T., & Kaplan, J. R. (1989). Psychophysiologic reactivity as a dimension of individual differences. In N. Schneiderman, S. M. Weiss, & P. G. Kaufmann (Eds.), *Handbook of research methods in cardiovascular behavioral medicine* (pp. 365–382). New York: Plenum.

Myrtek, M., & Foerster, F. (1986). The Law of Initial Values: A rare exception. *Biological Psychology, 22,* 227–237.

Porges, S. W., & Bohrer, R. E. (1990). The analysis of periodic processes in psychophysiological research. In J. T. Cacioppo & L. G. Tassinary (Eds.), *Principles of psychophysiology: Physical, social and inferential elements* (pp. 708–753). New York: Cambridge University Press.

Pritchard, W. S. & Duke, D. W. (1995). Measuring "chaos" in the brain: a tutorial review of EEG dimension estimation. *Brain and Cognition, 27,* 353–397.

Samar, V. J., Bopardikar, A., Rao, R., & Swartz, K. (1999). Wavelets: An application to human performance monitoring. *Brain & Language, 66,* 89–107.

Seraganian, P., Hanley, J. A., Hollander, B. J., Roskies, E., Smilga, C., Martin, N. D., Collu, R., & Oseasohn, R. (1985). Exaggerated psychophysiological reactivity: Issues in quantification and reliability. *Journal of Psychosomatic Research, 29,* 393–405.

Stern, J. A., & Dunham, D. N. (1990). The ocular system. In J. T. Cacioppo & L. G. Tassinary (Eds.), *Principles of psychophysiology: Physical, social, and inferential elements* (pp. 513–553). New York: Cambridge University Press.

Stern, R. M., Koch, K. L., & Vasey, M. W. (1990). The gastrointestinal system. In J. T. Cacioppo & L. G. Tassinary (Eds.). *Principles of psychophysiology: Physical, social, and inferential elements* (pp. 554–579). New York: Cambridge University Press.

Theiler, J. (1990) *Estimating the fractal dimension of chaotic time series.* Lincoln Laboratory Journal 3: 63–86.

Tomarken, A. J. (1995). A psychometric perspective on psychophysiological measures. *Psychological Assessment, 7,* 387–395.

# PART III

# *Applications*

# 15

## Applications of Psychophysiological Recording

Once an individual is able to record psychophysiological measures successfully, the question arises as to how these measures might be used in understanding the interdependence between psychological and physiological processes. What fields of study might significantly benefit from psychophysiological approaches?

Before beginning a discussion of applications of psychophysiological recording, we wish to refer back to some of the principles of psychophysiology introduced in chapter 5. Researchers have at times ignored these principles—these complexities—and have attempted to place such concepts as emotionality or arousal along a continuum. These same researchers would then try in vain to find a single physiological measure that would show a high correlation with a given psychophysiological concept. These simplistic studies were performed even in the midst of more appropriate conceptualizations of psychophysiological functioning. For example, in his review of psychophysiological approaches to the evaluation of psychotherapy outcome, Lacey (1959) emphasized that no one measure of bodily arousal was adequate in relation to either psychological process variables or other physiological measures. In this review and elsewhere, Lacey (as well as other pioneers Chester Darrow, and R. C. Davis) suggested that there are patterns of psychophysiological responding. This patterning is related to both the type of external stimuli (either sensory or "ideational," in Darrow's terminology, or "stimulus response specificity" in Lacey's) and the individual's physiological response pattern, which Lacey referred to as individual response stereotypy. Although Darrow (1929) presented his conceptualizations more than seventy years ago, today one still sees researchers attempting to use a single psychophysiological measure as an indicant of emotionality and arousal without regard to either situational or individual variables. With this cautionary note, let us now examine some examples of recent psychophysiological research.

## Five Categories of Psychophysiological Studies

If one were to review the journal *Psychophysiology* as well as books in psychophysiology one could divide psychophysiological studies into those that emphasize any one of five separate aspects. These categories are not seen as mutually exclusive or all inclusive but are presented here to offer an organizing principle for discussing recent psychophysiological research. These approaches, or emphases, are: (1) response variables, (2) stimulus/situational variables, (3) subject variables, (4) correlational variables, and (5) the applications of psychophysiological research.

### Response Variables

These studies are primarily concerned with properties of the psychophysiological response. Examples include examining the relation between electroencephalogram (EEG) alpha activity and metabolic activity in the thalamus, because EEG alpha activity has been thought to be modulated by the thalamus (Larson et al., 1998); neuroanatomical correlates of electrodermal activity (Fredrikson et al., 1998), the study of pulse wave transit time and its relationship to blood pressure (Steptoe, Smulyan, & Gribbin, 1976); ways of measuring the psychophysiological response, as in the case of frontalis EMG placements (Davis, Brickett, Stern, & Kimball, 1978); problems of instrumentation, as in the effect of time constants on the evoked potential P300 component (Duncan-Johnson & Donchin, 1979); problems of interpretation and quantification, as in the differences in heart rate and heart period measurements (Graham, 1978; Quigley & Berntson, 1996); and methods of statistical analysis using more than one occurrence or more than one psychophysiological measure (Vasey & Thayer, 1987). From its beginning in 1964, *Psychophysiology* has considered these questions to be at the heart of psychophysiological research and the journal includes a separate section for advances in instrumentation as well as methodology.

### Stimulus/Situational Variables

Studies that emphasize stimulus/situational variables are generally designed to examine differential psychophysiological responding as a function of different types of stimuli, either internal or external to the individual. These studies predate the formal study of psychophysiology and are among the first psychological studies of the last century. For example, in 1888 Féré published a report on the effects of stimuli such as colored glasses, the sounds of tuning forks, and stimuli involving taste and smell on electrodermal responses (Féré, 1888/1976). C. G. Jung, at the turn of the twentieth century, noted the electrodermal response to various emotionally arousing and neutral words. Other studies noted the effects of music on heart rate and respiration. In the twentieth century, Darrow (1929) reviewed the research concerning psychophysiological reactions to ideational and sensory stimuli. This tradition has been continued by a variety of researchers (e.g., Ray & Cole, 1985; Turpin, 1986).

## Subject Variables

Studies that examine these variables emphasize particular characteristics of the subjects themselves. These characteristics may be subdivided into five general classes: (1) state factors, (2) trait factors, (3) psychopathological factors, (4) organizational factors, and (5) evolving factors. State variables emphasize certain naturally occurring states within the individual. One commonly researched state factor is sleep. For example, Burgess, Kleiman, and Trinder (1999) examined cardiac activity during sleep onset; McDonald, Shallenberger, Kortesko, and Kinzy (1976) recorded spontaneous electrodermal responses during sleep. Other studies have looked at such states as hypnosis (e.g., Graffin, Ray, & Lundy, 1995; Dumas, 1977; Hilgard et al., 1974), and menstrual cycle (e.g., Little & Zahn, 1974; see Bell, Christie, & Venables, 1975, for a review of this area).

Trait or personality factors emphasize those characteristics of an individual which are seen as persisting in a variety of situations. One approach has been to examine psychophysiological variables in twins. An example of this work would be an examination of EEG characteristics in monozygotic and dizygotic twins (Christian et al., 1996). Other studies have examined individual difference characteristics such as hostility (Sul & Wan, 1993), locus of control (Ray, 1974), stimulation seeking (Zuckerman, Murtaugh, and Siegel, 1974), and anxiety (Heller, Nitschke, Etienne, & Miller, 1997; Neary and Zuckerman, 1976).

Underlying many of the specific studies of personality or trait variables are the numerous theories of personality types, such as that of Jung (1971) who in 1920 divided people into thinking, feeling, sensing, and intuitive types; Eysenck (1953), who classified people in terms of neuroticism and introversion/extroversion; and Pavlov (1928), who discussed temperaments in terms of Hippocrates' four types (i.e., choleric, melancholic, sanguine, and phlegmatic). All of these theories had implications for psychophysiological research. In the last part of the twentieth century, measures of personality involving the "Big Five" (extraversion, neuroticism, openness, agreeableness, and conscientiousness) have become the standard measure of individual differences and are sparking a variety of psychophysiological studies.

The third class of subject variables is the psychopathological or physiopathological factors. In studies emphasizing these factors, subjects are divided according to some preestablished diagnostic system, such as the *Diagnostic and statistical manual of mental disorders* (4th ed.) (DSM) (APA, 1994). These systems include both psychological disorders such as schizophrenia (Clementz, 1996; Rößner, Rockstroh, Cohen, Wagner, & Elbert, 1999; Yee, Nuechterlein, & Dawson, 1998) and psychopathy (Blackburn, 1979; Raskin and Hare, 1978; Williamson, Harpur, & Hare, 1991), as well as physiological disorders such as ulcers, hypertension, and headaches (Shapiro, Jammer, & Goldstein, 1997). The task of the psychophysiological researcher is to determine the important parameters of the psychological-physiological interface. One approach is to examine individuals who are unable to identify or communicate affective experiences (Roedema & Simons, 1999).

A fourth category is that of organizational differences, including such variables as race and gender. Although most psychophysiological studies have been performed with Caucasians who are male, there is evidence to suggest that both race and gender play a role in differential psychophysiological responding (Vrana & Rollock, 1998). Electrodermal activity in a variety of studies has been shown to be sensitive to racial differences (cf. Fisher & Kotses, 1973; James, Worland, and Stern, 1976; Lieblich, Kugelmass, and Ben-Shakhar, 1973), as has the electrogastrogram (EGG) (e.g., Stern, Breen, Watanabe, & Perry, 1996). Likewise, gender differences have been shown to be a significant variable in a number of psychophysiological studies (e.g., Beaumont & Mayes, 1977; Davidson & Schwartz, 1976; Heiman, 1977; Ketterer & Smith, 1977; Ray, Morell, Frediani, & Tucker, 1976). Both race and gender variables are extremely relevant in attempting to understand how hormonal, nervous system, and experimental influences interact to produce the observed psychophysiological response.

We refer to the fifth class of subject variables to as evolving factors. This category includes studies that examine a psychophysiological variable as it evolves over time. The clearest example of this type of research is psychophysiological studies within the area of lifespan development. So far, research in this area has focused on the differences between the electrophysiological responding of older and younger individuals. For example, Morgan Geisler, Covington, Polich, & Murphy (1999) examined event-related potential differences in young (age 20s) and older (age 60s) adults. The examination of age differences in EEG dates back to the 1930s and the work of Hans Berger. Other psychophysiological research has attempted to determine psychophysiological responses in the developing human organism. For example, Schaefer (1975) used EEG to examine neonatal responses to external stimulation; Graham and Jackson (1970) have used heart rate measures.

## Correlational Variables

For many researchers, these factors are both the most interesting to discuss and the most difficult to study. They are interesting to discuss because they include such traditional philosophical issues as the mind-brain question and the relation of bodily change to emotion and behavior. But, they are difficult to research because, by definition, these studies attempt to understand activity on one level of human activity from its correlation with activity on another level. The most commonly used classification of activity levels is a modern version of the Platonic organization presented in chapter 1. The modern version divides psychological activity into (1) cognitive activity, which may include so-called higher activity such as creativity, awareness, and consciousness; (2) emotional activity; and (3) instinctual activity. Whereas the psychological researcher correlates activity from one of these three levels with the other, the psychophysiological researcher correlates each with physiological responding. Psychophysiology offers researchers a window into cognitive and emotional processing. One fruitful area has been the study of cognition and attention (see Osman, 1998, for an overview). Another area has been that of language processing, particularly the use of electrocortical measures to study language structure and expectation (see Kutas, 1997, for an overview).

Another example of this type of research is found in the area of brain lateralization and activation. Doyle, Ornstein, and Galin (1974) suggested that EEG power relationships between the two cerebral hemispheres could be used to differentiate different types of cognitive processing, such as linguistic versus spatial processing. In a similar vein, a variety of studies have suggested that EEG measures might also be related to the processing of negative or positive emotional material (Davidson, 1995). Other studies outside of the hemispheric paradigm have sought to discover correlations between the electrical activity of the brain and such concepts as creativity, altered states of consciousness, and meditative experiences. Psychophysiological correlations with instinctual activity such as sexuality have also been observed and recorded. Although there are many studies on the correlations of cognitive, emotional, and instinctual behavior with psychophysiological variables, both the basic physiological mechanisms and the philosophical questions concerning the similarities among these levels of analysis remain unresolved.

## Application Studies

The final category we will discuss includes those studies that attempt to understand psychophysiological principles as they are applied in real-world settings. Three examples these types of research are biofeedback, lie detection, and brain plasticity and pain.

*Biofeedback.* Until the 1960s, it was assumed that autonomic nervous system (ANS) responses had to be elicited rather than emitted, thus involving the procedures of classical conditioning. Central nervous system (CNS) responses, on the other hand, were considered to be voluntary and thus reinforced by the techniques of operant conditioning. These speculations were largely untested until Miller (1963) questioned the traditional differences between classical and operant conditioning. Miller suggested that there is really only one type of learning; classical and operant conditioning are two manifestations of the same phenomenon under different conditions. It follows that if there is only one type of learning, autonomic responses should be conditionable through operant methods. Thus, the 1960s saw a number of research studies directed at this question.

The initial studies were performed with animals. In order to demonstrate autonomic conditioning, it was first thought necessary to show that there was no somatic intervention. For example, if one wanted to condition the heart, it would be important to show that the heart rate changes were not due to respiratory changes. The control of somatic mediation was achieved by paralyzing the animal's CNS.

However, when working with human beings, the question became more difficult, as the reviews by Kimmel (1967) and Katkin and Murray (1968) point out. Not only was there a possibility of somatic mediation, but there was also the question of cognitive mediation. The question became how to conceptualize the situation in which arousing or angry thoughts produced a change in heart rate. Could this be considered an example of human autonomic conditioning? Although there was much debate, the question was never really answered.

The conditioning question was reformulated into a question of control. That is, rather than asking if autonomic conditioning were possible, researchers looked to find under what conditions an individual could demonstrate physiological self-control. Research in "operant conditioning" was replaced by an interest in "biofeedback." Biofeedback is a deceptively simple technique in which information from physiological responses such as EEG, muscle tension, and so forth is fed back to the individual, with the final goal being the self-regulation of the physiological function.

The transition from operant conditioning to biofeedback involved a movement from theory to practicality. Initial research questions focused on the type of feedback that was optimal and the importance of awareness in learning self-control. Clinical researchers suggested that the manner in which patients self-regulated their hypertension, for example, was less important than the possibility of returning their blood pressure to within normal limits. Biofeedback became the new panacea for a number of disorders including headaches, epilepsy, cardiac arrhythmias, and dental and neuromuscular disorders. However, 10 years after the first biofeedback studies, the therapeutic efficacy was still in question for a large number of disorders (Ray, Raczynski, Rogers, & Kimball, 1979) and remains so today. However, there are a number of success stories which make this work intriguing. For example, a variety of studies from the Tübingen lab of Niels Birbaumer reported that teaching epileptics to modify slow-wave EEG behavior resulted in a reduction of seizures. These studies were also performed with children with attentional disorders as well as healthy volunteers (see Rockstroh, Elber, Canavan, Lutzenberger, & Birbaumer, 1989 for a review). In these studies, slow-wave activity was recorded along the midline of the cortex. Changes in the EEG moved a symbolic rocket ship from left to right on a computer screen during a 6-s period. The task was to direct the rocket ship toward one of two locations on the screen through the generation or suppression of cortical negativity. The results from these studies suggest that individuals can learn to control slow cortical potentials in both a negative and positive direction within about 80 to 160 feedback trials. Another important use of EEG biofeedback technology has been to teach paralyzed individuals to communicate. Birbaumer and his colleagues describe the case of an individual completed paralyzed who was able to use his brain waves to slowly spell out words and communicate with the outside world (Birbaumer et al., 1999).

*Lie Detection.* Lie detection refers to a variety of procedures whereby ANS measures such as blood pressure, pulse rate, and electrodermal activity are recorded from an individual while the person is asked two types of questions: relevant and comparison. The relevant questions deal with specifics of a crime under investigation or some aspect of the individual's personal life. The latter variety are sometimes used in preemployment screening by government agencies that deal with security matters. The use of lie detection in preemployment screening by private companies has been outlawed in the United States.

Comparison questions are always included in the interrogation process in order to determine the magnitude of the individual's ANS responses in answering nonrelevant questions alone. As we discussed in chapter 5, individual responding using various psychophysiological measures varies greatly from person to person. Without this information, an individual might be falsely accused of being guilty or suppressing information just because of large ANS responses made to all questions.

The formulation of the questions to be asked a crime suspect or job applicant for a position in a governmental security agency is a highly technical and somewhat controversial matter. Raskin and his colleagues (e.g., Podlesny and Raskin, 1977) recommend the use of the control-question technique. The control questions (used instead of neutral questions), formulated during a pretest interview, are selected so that the individual will probably be deceptive or at least very concerned about them. An example of a control question used in a theft case would be, "During the first eighteen years of your life, did you ever steal something from someone who trusted you?" The rationale for this technique is explained by Podlesny and Raskin (1977): "The control question approach attempts to set up a situation wherein a subject who is truthful concerning relevant questions will be more concerned about the control questions and will produce greater responses to them than to the relevant questions. Similarly, deception on relevant questions should make the subject more responsive to relevant than to control questions" (p. 786). Another discussion of the control-question technique can be found in Honts, Kircher, and Raskin (1995). The interested reader is also referred to an article by Furedy (1996) in which he raises ethical problems that he claims are inherent in the use of the control-question method.

Lykken (1974, 1979, 1991) has questioned many of the claims and assumptions of proponents of traditional lie detection procedures such as the control-question test. According to Lykken, psychophysiological recordings cannot and should not be used to determine whether or not someone is lying. He suggests an alternative and related use, however. Lykken's procedure, referred to as the guilty-knowledge test, is based upon the presence or absence of differential responsivity to items of information that only the guilty suspect would recognize as being relevant. If the person being questioned did not murder the girl in the red dress, a question about red dresses should bring about ANS responses no larger than responses to a question about blue dresses.

We believe that there are two assumptions that must be examined in order to test the validity of any of these procedures. The first assumption is that lying (or possessing guilty knowledge) will cause heightened ANS responding. This is true for most but not all individuals. The second assumption is that the ANS responses used in the lie detection procedure are not under the suspect's voluntary control. This assumption is more questionable, particularly in light of work in the area of biofeedback (see chapter 20 in Stern & Ray, 1977). It should be noted that individuals can learn, through the use of biofeedback over many trials, to control their ANS responses, but when participants are provided with feedback of their physiological responses during an interrogation, they are easier to detect than subjects in a no-feedback control group (Stern, Breen, Watanabe, & Perry, 1981).

The psychophysiological response measures used in lie detection situations are more relevant to this book than are the interrogation procedures. The following response variables have been used in laboratory and field tests: respiration, blood pressure, electrodermal activity, pulse rate, pulse volume, muscular tension, eye movement, and eye blinks. Curiously, in laboratory tests, electrodermal activity is usually the best single indicator of deception, but in actual field use, the cardiovascular measures discriminate best. This apparent discrepancy may be a function of basic differences in laboratory and field situations. These differences include level of emotional involvement of the subjects and differences between the background and training of the people doing the interrogating. Laboratory lie detection studies are usually conducted by psychologists interested in psychophysiology. Field testing in lie detection is usually done by individuals with a background in police work. These two groups of investigators not only have different backgrounds and goals but also use different equipment and recording techniques. They have a lot to offer each other but, unfortunately, few individuals belong to both the American Polygraph Association and to scientific psychological research societies.

Lie detection raises a number of important questions for psychophysiologists to consider. Some of these questions are as follows:

1. Does a person's physiology actually mirror that person's state of emotional arousal?
2. Can we differentiate between increases in emotional arousal caused by lying versus other states such as worry or embarrassment?
3. Are there some individuals, such as psychopaths, for whom we cannot use the lie detector?
4. Can a person, through biofeedback or other techniques, learn to modify his physiological responding and thus "fool" a lie detection operator?
5. To what extent can augmented physiological feedback aid in the detection of deception?
6. What does traditional theory in psychophysiology concerning habituation, sensitization, motivation, stimulus presentation, arousal, and so forth have to offer the field of lie detection, and vice versa?

Lie detection has received only minor interest by psychophysiologists, the result being little long-term systematic research in the area. Yet as an area with both applied and theoretical implications, it appears to offer the psychophysiological researcher numerous opportunities and challenges. For a bibliography of lie detection, see Ansley and Horvath (1977). Other reviews that may be consulted include Davis (1961) and Orne, Thackray, and Paskewitz (1972).

*Cognitive Neuroscience:* Cognitive neuroscience is a multileveled approach to the understanding of the mind, including cognitive, emotional, and motor processes. Psychophysiology has emerged as an important tool that aids researchers and clinicians in describing the underlying mechanisms in both normal and pathological functions. In this section we will sample a variety of cognitive areas that have made use of psychophysiological techniques.

Cortical plasticity and reorganization after injury is one area that has used psychophysiological approaches, especially brain mapping techniques, to obtain a better understanding of brain processes. If a person is in an accident that results in the removal of an arm or leg, the area of the brain that was associated with bodily sensation and movement of that limb changes and reorganizes itself in a new way. Using magnetoencephalogram (MEG) techniques, Ramachandran and his colleagues (see Ramachandran & Hirstein, 1998, for a review) described four individuals who had their arms amputated. In all four individuals, these researchers found that the area of the cortex associated with the hand changed to become associated with the face and upper arm. In fact, if a cotton swab was lightly rubbed on one individual's lower face, he reported feeling sensations in the missing arm. Likewise, warm water trickling down the face would be experienced both on the face and down the length of the missing arm. Given that a traumatic experience such as losing an arm could cause cortical reorganization, one could also ask if normal experience itself could have an influence. The answer to this question turns out to be yes. Using MEG techniques, Elbert and his colleagues compared string players who had played instruments throughout their lives with a group of controls (Elbert, Panter, Wienbruch, Rockstroh, & Taub, 1995). Not only was the cortical representation of the fingers of the left hand of string players larger than that in controls, but the amount of cortical reorganization in the representation of the fingering digits was correlated with the age at which the person had begun to play.

Another area that has benefited from psychophysiological techniques is that of attention. An interesting question in attention is how we pick out one aspect of the multitude of sounds, images, sensations, and so on that constantly confront us (see Luck, 1998 for an overview of this question). A great variety of ERP studies have been performed to determine when particular types of information are processed in the cortex. For example, Hillyard and colleagues (1973) studied the influence of attending or not attending to a particular stimulus. They found that when one attends to a stimulus, the first negative component (N1) of the ERP is larger than when one did not. Since this N1 component peaks at approximately 100 ms after a stimulus presentation, these researchers concluded that selective attention acts at a very early stage of processing. Another type of attention research has examined if deaf or blind individuals have enhanced capabilities of sensory processing. For example, Röder and colleagues (1999) report a differential pattern of N1 activity across the scalp in individuals who are blind versus sighted individuals with a blindfold. They also reported localization abilities of blind individuals to be superior to sighted ones, but only when the stimuli were presented in the periphery.

As we look at an object, we see it as a whole even through various aspects of it (color, smell, taste, texture, complexity, etc.) are encoded and processed in different parts of the brain. This question has come to be called the "binding" question in that it asks how the brain puts or binds together various aspects of an experience to produce a coherent whole. One answer to this question has come from EEG research. A variety of studies have shown that oscillatory synchronization of the EEG in the gamma band (30–80 Hz) is associated with feature binding in a variety of modalities including vision (see Singer & Gray, 1995; Tallon-Baudry & Bertrand, 1999, for a review of this work). Using EEG measures and wavelet analysis, Tallon-Baudry and her colleagues showed enhanced gamma band activity when an individual recognized a hidden figure (a Dalmatian dog) but not when the figure appeared as meaningless black blobs on a grey background. Likewise, Keil Müller, Ray, Gruber, & Elbert (1999) showed enhanced gamma band activity when an ambiguous figure (either a happy or sad face depending on orientation) switched to a new perspective. Using classical conditioning to establish a relationship between a visual and tactile stimulus, Miltner Braun, Witte, & Taub (1999) showed greater EEG gamma band coherence between areas in the brain that are involved in visual and tactile experiences. Once the conditioning relationship between the visual and tactile stimuli was extinguished, the EEG coherence decreased.

In each of the areas discussed—cortical reorganization, attention, and binding—psychophysiological techniques helped to answer questions concerning temporal and spatial aspects of the process. In these examples, the evoked potential was particularly important for understanding when certain types of processing took place, whereas the brain mapping techniques were useful for describing which areas were involved in a particular activity. Other areas of research, such as motor processing and emotional experience and expression, have also benefited from psychophysiological studies; the interested student should consult such journals as *Psychophysiology* for reports of recent work.

## Conclusions

With the availability of small laboratory computers and newer instruments for the recording of physiological measures, it is clear that we will see an increasing number of psychophysiological studies being performed in traditional areas of psychology. We also predict an increase in real-world applications of psychophysiology as greater use is made of telemetry, ambulatory recordings, and nonintrusive recording techniques (Fahrenberg & Myrtek, 1996). As mentioned previously, psychophysiological studies in the area of lifespan development, especially aging and neonatal development, are beginning to increase in both number and sophistication. Other areas, such as biofeedback and behavioral medicine, sleep, and pain, are continuing to draw the interest of researchers and clinicians who can make significant contributions based on their understanding of psychophysiological principles.

Just as psychophysiologists are able to contribute to new and developing areas, they must also be ready to integrate new aspects of these areas into their research. For example, the standard statistical procedure of determining significance through the use of techniques such as analysis of variance may be combined with newer nonlinear models of human functioning. For example, researchers in the area of behavioral medicine ask how a number of treatment techniques can combine to form a sum greater than any of the parts alone. Likewise, developmental studies demonstrate the importance of certain changes of physiological state (e.g., puberty) that result in irreversible processes impossible to discuss from a simple acquisition and extinction paradigm.

We end this book as we began. In the beginning, we indicated that psychophysiology had a short history and a long past. We described the subject matter of psychophysiology as not new but as represented by broad questions studied for centuries by individuals trained as philosophers, physicists, physicians, physiologists, and psychologists. We would like to point out that as the name implies, psychophysiology is at the heart of one of the most fascinating and enduring of these issues: the relationship between mind and body. It is our hope that with the aid of psychophysiological recording you will gain insights into the basic nature of this and other fundamental questions.

### References

American Psychiatric Association. (1994). *Diagnostic and statistical manual of mental disorders* (4th ed.). Washington, DC: Author.

Ansley, N., & Horvath, F. (1977). *Truth and science: A comprehensive index to international literature on the detection of deception and the polygraph (lie detector) technique.* Linthicum Heights, MD: American Polygraph Association.

Beaumont, G., & Mayes, A. (1977). Do task and sex differences influence the visual evoked potential? *Psychophysiology, 14.* 545–550.

Bell, B., Christie, M. J., & Venables, P. H. (1975). Psychophysiology of the menstrual cycle. In P. H. Venables & M. J. Christie (Eds.), *Research in psychophysiology.* London: Wiley.

Birbaumer, N., Ghanayim, N., Hinterberger, T., Iversen, I., Kotchoubey, B., Kübler, A., Perelmouter, J., Taub, E., & Flor, H. (1999) A spelling device for the paralysed. *Nature, 398,* 297–298.

Blackburn, R. (1979). Cortical and autonomic arousal in primary and secondary psychopaths. *Psychophysiology, 16,* 143–150.

Burgess, H., Kleiman, J., & Trinder, J. (1999) Cardiac activity during sleep onset. *Psychophysiology, 36,* 298–306.

Christian, J., Morzorati, S., Norton, J., Williams, C., O onnor, S., & Li, T. (1996) Genetic analysis of the resting electroencephalographic power spectrum in human twins. *Psychophysiology, 33*, 584–591.

Clementz, B. (1996). Saccades to moving targets in schizophrenia: Evidence for normal posterior cortex functioning. *Psychophysiology, 33*, 650–654.

Darrow, C. W. (1929). Differences in the physiological reactions to sensory and ideational stimuli. *Psychological Bulletin, 26*, 185–201.

Davidson, R. J. (1995). Cerebral asymmetry, emotion, and affective style. In R. J. Davidson & K. Hugdahl (Eds.), *Brain Asymmetry* (361–387). Cambridge, MA: MIT Press.

Davidson, R. J., & Schwartz, G. E. (1976). Patterns of cerebral lateralization during cardiac biofeedback versus the self-regulation of emotion: Sex differences. *Psychophysiology, 13*, 62–68.

Davis, C. M., Brickett, P., Stern, R. M., & Kimball, W. H. (1978). Tension in two frontales: Electrode placement and artifact in the recording of the forehead EMG. *Psychophysiology, 15*, 591–593.

Davis, R. C. (1961). Physiological responses as a means of evaluating information. In A. Biderman and H. Zimmet (Eds.), *Manipulation of human behavior*. New York: Wiley.

Doyle, J. C., Ornstein, R., & Galin, D. (1974). Lateral specialization of cognitive mode: II. EEG frequency analysis. *Psychophysiology, 11*, 567–578.

Dumas, R. A. (1977). EEG alpha-hynotizability correlations: A review. *Psychophysiology, 14*, 431–438.

Duncan-Johnson, C. C., & Donchin, E. (1979). The time constant in P300 recording. *Psychophysiology, 16*, 53–55.

Elbert, T., Pantev, C., Wienbruch, C., Rockstroh, B., & Taub, E. (1995). Increased cortical representation of the fingers of the left hand in string players. *Science, 270*, 305–307

Eysenck, H. J. (1953). *The structure of human personality*. New York: Wiley.

Fahrenberg, J., & Myrtek, M. (Eds.)(1996) *Ambulatory Assessment*. Seattle: Hogrefe & Huber Publishers.

Féré, C. (1888/1976) (Note of changes in electrical resistance under the effect of sensory stimulation and emotion). In S. W. Porges and M. G. H. Coles (Eds.), *Psychophysiology*. Stroudsburg, PA: Dowden, Hutchinson & Ross.

Fisher, L. E., & Kotses, H. (1973). Race differences and experimenter race effect in galvanic skin response. *Psychophysiology, 10*, 578–582.

Fredrikson, M., Furmark, T., Olsson, M., Fischer, H., Andersson, J., & Långström, B. (1998) Functional neuroanatomical correlates of electrodermal activity: A positron emission tomographic study. *Psychophysiology, 35*, 179–185.

Furedy, J. J. (1996). Some elementary distinctions among, and comments concerning, the "control" question "test" (CQT) polygrapher's many problems: A reply to Honts, Kircher, and Raskin. *International Journal of Psychophysiology, 22*, 53–59.

Galin, D., & Ornstein, R. (1972). Lateral specialization of cognitive mode: An EEG study. *Psychophysiology, 9*, 412–418.

Graffin, N., Ray, W., & Lundy, R. (1995) EEG concomitants of hypnosis and hypnotic susceptibility, *Journal of Abnormal Psychology, 104*, 123–131.

Graham, F. K. (1978). Normality of distributions and homogeneity of variance of heart rate and heart period samples. *Psychophysiology, 15*, 487–491.

Graham, F., & Jackson, J. C. (1970). Arousal systems and infant heart rate responses. In H. W. Reese & L. P. Lipsitt (Eds.), *Advances in child development and behavior*. New York: Academic Press.

Heiman, J. R. (1977). A psychophysiological exploration of sexual arousal patterns in females and males. *Psychophysiology, 14*, 266–274.

Heller, W., Nitschke, J. B., Etienne, M. A., & Miller, G. A. (1997). Patterns of regional brain activity differentiate types of anxiety. *Journal of Abnormal Psychology, 106*, 376–385.

Hilgard, E., Morgan, A. H., Lange, A. F., Lenox, J. R., MacDonald, H., & Marshall, G. (1974). Heart rate changes in pain and hypnosis. *Psychophysiology, 11*, 692–702.

Hillyard, S., Hink, R., Schwent, V., & Picton, T. (1973) Electrical signs of selective attention in the human brain. *Science, 182*, 177–179.

Honts, C. R., Kircher, J. C., & Raskin, D. C. (1995). Polygrapher's dilemma or psychologist's chimaera: A reply to Furedy's logico-ethical considerations for psychophysiological practitioners and researchers. *International Journal of Psychophysiology, 20*, 199–207.

James, C. L., Worland, J., & Stern, J. (1976). Skin potential and vasomotor responsiveness of black and white children. *Psychophysiology, 13*, 523–527.

Jung, C. G. (1971). *Psychological types*. Princeton, N. J.; Princeton University Press.

Katkin, E. S., & Murray, E. N. (1968). Instrumental conditioning of autonomic mediated behavior: Theoretical and methodological issues. *Psychological Bulletin, 70*, 52–68.

Keil, A., Müller, M., Ray, W., Gruber, T., & Elbert, T. (1999) Human gamma band activity and perception of a gestalt. *Journal of Neuroscience, 19*, 7152–7161.

Ketterer, M. W., & Smith, B. D. (1977). Bilateral electrical activity, lateralized cerebral processing and sex. *Psychophysiology, 14*, 513–516.

Kimmel, H. D. (1967). Instrumental conditioning of autonomically mediated behavior. *Psychological Bulletin, 67*, 337–345.

Kutas, M. (1997) Views on how the electrical activity that the brain generates reflects the functions of different language structures. *Psychophysiology, 34*, 383–398.

Lacey, J. I. (1959). Psychophysiological approaches to the evaluation of psychotherapeutic process and outcome. In E. A. Rubenstein and M. B. Parloff (Eds.), *Research in psychotherapy* (Vol. 1). Washington, D. C.: American Psychological Association.

Larson, C., Davidson, R., Abercrombie, H., Ward, R., Schaefer, S., Jackson, D., Holden, J., & Perlman, S. (1998). Relations between PET-derived measures of thalamic glucose metabolism and EEG alpha power. *Psychophysiology, 35*, 162–169.

Lieblich, I., Kugelmass, S., & Ben-Shakhar, G. (1973). Psychophysiological baselines as a function of race and ethnic origin. *Psychophysiology, 10*, 426–430.

Little, B. C., & Zahn, T. P. (1974). Changes in mood and autonomic functioning during the menstrual cycle. *Psychophysiology, 11*, 579–590.

Luck, S. (1998). Neurophysiology of selective attention. In H. Pashler (Ed.), *Attention*. East Sussex, UK: Psychology Press.

Lykken, D. T. (1974). Psychology and the lie detector industry. *American Psychologist, 29*, 725–739.

Lykken, D. T. (1979). The detection of deception. *Psychological Bulletin, 10*, 166–176.

Lykken, D. T. (1991). Why (some) Americans believe in the lie detector while others believe in the guilty knowledge test. *Integrated Physiology and Behavioral Science, 26*, 214–222.

McDonald, D. G., Shallenberger, H. D., Koresko, R. L., and Kinzy, B. G. (1976). Studies of spontaneous electrodermal responses in sleep. *Psychophysiology, 13*, 128–134.

Miller, N (1963) Some reflections on the law of effect produce a new alternative to drive reduction. In R. Jones (Eds.), *Nebraska symposium on motivation*. Lincoln, NE: University of Nebraska Press.

Miltner, W., Braun, C., Witte, A., & Taub, E. (1999). Coherence of gamma-band EEG activity as a basis for associative learning. *Nature, 397*, 434–436.

Morgan, C., Geisler, M., Covington, J., Polich, J., & Murphy, C. (1999) Olfactory P3 in young and older adults. *Psychophysiology, 36*, 281–287.

Neary, R., and Zukerman, M. (1976). Sensation seeking trait and state anxiety, and the electrodermal orienting response. *Psychophysiology, 13*, 205–211.

Orne, M. T., Thackray, R. I., & Paskewitz, D. A. (1972). On the detection of deception: A model for the study of the physiological effects of psychological stimuli. In N. S. Greenfield and R. A. Sternbach, (Eds.), *Handbook of psychophysiology*. New York: Holt, Reinhart & Winston.

Osman, A. (1998). Brainwaves and mental processes: Electrical evidence of attention, perception, and intention. In D. Scarborough and S. Sternberg (Eds.) *Methods, Models, and Conceptual Issues*. Cambridge, MA: MIT Press.

Pavlov, I. P. (1928). *Lectures on conditioned reflexes. Vol. 1*. W. H. Gantt (Ed. and trans.). New York: International Publishers.

Podlesny, J. A., & Raskin, D. C. (1977). Physiological measures and the detection of deception. *Psychological Bulletin, 84*, 782–799.

Pritchard, W., Robinson, J., deBethizy, J., Davis, R., & Stiles, M. (1995) Caffeine and smoking: Subjective, performance, and psychophysiological effects. *Psychophysiology, 32*, 19–27.

Quigley, K., & Berntson, G. (1996) Autonomic interactions and chronotropic control of the heart: Heart period versus heart rate. *Psychophysiology, 33*, 605–611.

Ramachandran, V., & Hirstein, W. (1998). The perception of phantom limbs: The D. O. Hebb lecture. *Brain, 121*, 1603–1630.

Raskin, D. C., & Hare, R. D. (1978). Psychopathy and detection of deception in a prison population. *Psychophysiology, 15*, 126–136.

Raskin, D. C., Honts, C. R., & Kircher, J. C. (1997). Polygraph techniques: Theory, research, and applications from the perspective of scientists-practioners. In D. L. Faigman, D. Kaye, M. J. Saks, & J. Sanders (Eds.), *Scientific evidence reference manual*. St. Paul, MN: West Publishing Co.

Ray, W. J. (1974). The relationship of locus of control, self-report measures, and feedback to the voluntary control of heart rate. *Psychophysiology, 11*, 527–534.

Ray, W. J., Morell, M., Frediani, A., & Tucker, D. (1976). Sex differences and lateral specialization of hemispheric functioning. *Neuropsychologia, 14,* 391–394.

Ray, W. J., & Cole, H. W. (1985). EEG alpha reflects attentional demands, Beta reflects emotional and cognitive processes. *Science, 228,* 750–752.

Ray, W. J., Raczynski, J., Rogers, T., & Kimball, W. H. (1979). *Evaluation of clinical biofeedback.* New York: Plenum.

Rockstroh, B., Elber, T., Canavan, A., Lutzenberger, W., & Birbaumer, N. (1989). *Slow cortical potentials and behaviour.* Baltimore: Urban & Schwarzenberg.

Roedema, T., & Simons, R. (1999) Emotion-processing deficit in alexithymia. *Psychophysiology, 36,* 379–387.

Röder, B., Teder-Sälejärvi, W., Sterr, A., Rösler, F., Hillyard, S., & Neville, H. (1999). Improved auditory spatial tuning in blind humans. *Nature, 400,* 162–166.

Rößner, P., Rockstroh, B., Cohen, R., Wagner, M., & Elbert, T. (1999) Event-related potential correlates of proactive interference in schizophrenic patients and controls. *Psychophysiology, 36,* 199–208.

Schaefer, A. B. (1975). Newborn responses to non-signal auditory stimuli: I. Electroencephalographic desynchronization. *Psychophysiology, 12,* 673–681.

Shapiro, D., Jammer, L., & Goldstein, I. (1997) Daily mood states and ambulatory blood pressure. *Psychophysiology, 34,* 1997.

Singer, W., & Gray, C. (1995). Visual feature integration and the temporal correlation hypothesis. *Annual Review of Neuroscience, 18,* 555–586.

Steptoe, A., Smulyan, H., & Gribbin, B. (1976). Pulse wave velocity and blood pressure change: Calibration and applications. *Psychophysiology, 13,* 488–493.

Stern, R. M., Breen, J. P., Watanabe, T., & Perry, B. S. (1981). Effect of feedback of physiological information on responses to innocent associations and guilty knowledge. *Journal of Applied Psychology 66,* 677–681.

Stern, R. M., Hu, S., Uijtdehaage, S. H. J., Muth, E. R., Xu, L. H., & Koch, K. L. (1996). Asian hypersusceptibility to motion sickness. *Human Heredity, 46,* 7–14.

Stern, R. M., & Ray, W. J. (1980). *Biofeedback: Potential and limitations.* Lincoln, Ne: University of Nebraska Press.

Sul, J., & Wan, C. (1993) The relationship between trait hostility and cardiovascular reactivity: A quantitative review and analysis. *Psychophysiology, 30,* 615–626.

Tallon-Baudry, C., & Bertrand, O. (1999). Oscillatory gamma activity in humans and its role in object representation. *Trends in Cognitive Sciences, 3,* 151–162.

Turpin, G. (1986). Effects of stimulus intensity on autonomic responding: The problem of differentiating orienting and defensive reflexes. *Psychophysiology, 23,* 1–14.

Vasey, M., & Thayer, J. (1987) The continuing problem of false positives in repeated measures ANOVA in psychophysiology: A multivariate solution. *Psychophysiology, 24,* 479,486.

Vrana, S., & Rollock, D. (1998) Physiological response to a minimal social encounter: Effects of gender, ethnicity, and social context. *Psychophysiology, 35,* 462–469.

Williamson, S., Harpur, T., & Hare, R. (1991) Abnormal processing of affective words by psychopaths. *Psychophysiology, 28,* 260–273.

Woodruff, D. (1978). Brain electrical activity and behavior relationships over the life span. In P. Baltes (Ed.), *Life span development and behavior Vol. 1.* New York: Academic Press.

Yee, C., Nuechterlein, K., & Dawson, M. (1999) A longitudinal analysis of eye tracking dysfunction and attention in recent-onset schizophrenia. *Psychophysiology, 35,* 443–451.

Zuckerman, M. (1972). Physiological measure of sexual arousal in the human. In N. S. Greenfield and R. A. Sternbach (Eds.), *Handbook of psychophysiology.* New York: Holt, Reinhart & Winston.

Zuckerman, M., Murtagh, T., & Siegel, J. (1974). Sensation seeking and cortical augmenting-reducing. *Psychophysiology, 11,* 535–542.

# Glossary

*Acetylcholine:* neurotransmitter at all parasympathetic postganglionic and all preganglionic peripheral synapses and at the neuromuscular junction.

*Actin:* contractile protein in muscle fibrils; functions in conjunction with myosin.

*Action Potential:* sequence of changes in potential associated with impulse conduction in nerves and muscles.

*Adrenaline: see* Epinephrine.

*Adrenal Medulla:* portion of the adrenal gland which secretes epinephrine.

*Aliasing:* faulty representation of a digitized analog signal due to an insufficient sampling rate; an aliased signal will contain spurious frequency components that are not present in the original analog signal and will not contain some higher frequency components present in the original signal.

*Alpha Blocking:* the change in the EEG from alpha to other rhythms, usually beta.

*Alpha Rhythm:* relatively large, rhythmic brain waves of approximately 8–12 Hz, as recorded in an EEG; thought to be related to relaxation.

*Analog signal:* a continuous physiological signal.

*Analog-to-Digital (A-D) Converter:* device which converts a continuous physiological signal into discrete steps, enabling a computer to quantify the data.

*Antrum:* lower part of the stomach, from which EGG is recorded.

*Arousal:* often used synonymously with activation.

*Artifact:* stray and unwanted electrical signal in a physiological recording.

*Atrioventricular Node (A-V Node):* a small area of electrically active muscle in the right atria in which excitatory impulses arriving from the sinoatrial node are passed along to the conducting system of the heart.

*Auditory Evoked Response:* A predictable series of brain wave forms and distribution following each of a series of sounds; of maximum amplitude over the vertex of the brain.

*Autocorrelation:* the correlation between a digitized physiological record and itself lagged by some time period.

*Autonomic Lability Score (ALS):* a method of standardizing phasic ANS scores.

*Autonomic Nervous System (ANS):* ganglia, nerves, and plexuses which regulate activities of the viscera, heart, blood vessels, smooth muscle, and glands.

*Autoregulation:* one factor which increases the rate of blood flow during exercise; it responds to the local nutritional needs of the body.

*Axon:* neuron fiber processes that generally conduct impulses away from the cell body; long neuron fibers.

*Band-pass Filter:* a combination of a highpass and a lowpass filter set so that only a certain range of frequencies can pass.

*Baroreceptors:* sensory receptors found predominantly in the large arteries which detect changes in pressure when deformed.

*Beta Rhythm:* rhythmic brain waves of approximately 13–30 Hz, as recorded in an EEG, most often observed when the subject is alert.

*Biofeedback:* information concerning the functioning of internal organs, usually obtained through the use of electronic recording equipment.

*Bioelectric Potential:* a difference in electrical potential as recorded from different parts of a living organism.

*Bipolar Recording:* a recording method involving no reference electrode but rather a comparison of two active sites.

*Blood Volume:* a measure of the relatively slow changes in the amount of blood in an arm, finger, or other body structure.

*Bradygastria:* an abnormally slow rate of contractions of the stomach.

*Brain Stem Evoked Response (BSER):* an evoked response which originates in the brain stem area.

*Bucking Voltage:* an off-setting voltage used to neutralize an undesirable standing potential.

*Capacitance:* the property that permits a body or circuit to store an electrical charge; is equal to the stored charge divided by the voltage, and is expressed in farads.

*Cardiac Output (CO):* the amount of blood circulated through the body per unit of time (usually in liters/minute).

*Cardiac-somatic Coupling:* influence of motor activity on cardiovascular activity.

*Cardiotachometer:* a device for measuring heart rate that electronically determines the time from one QRS complex to the next and displays the information graphically in terms of beats per minute.

*Central Nervous System (CNS):* neural material contained in the spinal cord and brain.

*Chaos:* see nonlinear dynamical analysis

*Chemoreceptors:* sensory receptors sensitive to changes in the chemical milieu surrounding the receptor.

*Common Mode Rejection Ratio:* a measure of the ability of a differential amplifier to reject noise or interference.

*Compensatory Movement:* movement of the head or body in response to external movement.

*Contingent Negative Variation (CNV):* a slow negative potential, recorded in an EEG, typically occurring between a warning signal and a signal which instructs the subject to respond; similar to the readiness potential.

*Corneal-retinal Potential:* the potential between the cornea and retina of the eye; the basis of the EOG.

*Cortical:* describes a function or process associated with the cerebral cortex.

*Coupler:* used in the first stage of some polygraphs.

*Defensive Response:* pattern of responding which serves to limit action of a stimulus on an organism in order to protect the organism from possible dangers of intense stimulation.

*Delta Rhythm:* low EEG frequencies (0.5–4 Hz) associated with sleep.

*Dendrite:* neuron fiber processes that generally conduct impulses toward the cell body; short neuron fibers.

*Depolarization:* reduction or neutralization of polarity; typically occurs when the inside of an electrically excitable cell becomes less negative relative to the outside and therefore is closer to reaching threshold for initiating an action potential.

*Diastolic Blood Pressure (DBP):* the minimal pressure in the vascular system at the point where the measurement is taken; diastolic blood pressure occurs at the lowest point of the pressure pulse; units of millimeters of mercury (mmHg).

*Digital Filtering:* eliminates certain frequencies while others are allowed to pass.

*Digital signal:* a signal recreated from sequential, discrete samples of an analog physiological signal.

*Directional Fractionation:* a pattern of ANS responses characterized by some physiological responses suggestive of decreased arousal (e.g., a heart rate decrease) coupled with others suggestive of increased arousal (e.g., a skin conductance response).

*Eccrine Sweat Glands:* sweat glands, located primarily in the palms of hands and soles of feet, innervated by the sympathetic branch of the ANS; differ from other sweat glands because they respond primarily to "psychic" stimulation as opposed to increases in temperature.

*Electrical Control Activity (ECA):* basic electrical rhythm which controls the rhythmic contractions of the lower part of the stomach (antrum) by making the membrane temporarily susceptible to the generation of another potential i.e., the electrical response activity (ERA).

*Electrical Response Activity (ERA):* electrical potential consisting of one or more spikes superimposed on the decline phase of the electrical control activity (ECA) and preceding contractions of the lower portion of the stomach (antrum).

*Electrocardiography (EKG or ECG):* a technique for recording the electrical activity of the heart.

*Electrode:* conductor through which electricity enters or leaves a medium.

*Electrodermal Activity (EDA):* a measure of various electrical properties of the skin.

*Electroencephalography (EEG):* a technique for recording over time variations in electrical potentials observed from electrodes on the scalp.

*Electrogastrography (EGG):* a method for recording gastric myoelectric activity from the surface of the skin over the lower part of the stomach.

*Electrolyte:* a chemical compound, such as sodium chloride, that dissociates into ions when dissolved, forming a conductor.

*Electromyography (EMG):* a technique for recording the time, voltage graph of electrical potentials originating in muscles either from the surface of the skin (surface EMG) or from electrodes inserted into the muscle.

*Electrooculography (EOG):* a technique which records changes in the cornearetinal potential as a function of the movement of the eyes.

*Epinephrine (also called Adrenaline):* hormone secreted by the adrenal medulla which stimulates glucose production; acts on sympathetically innervated organs in a way similar to norepinephrine.

*Evoked Response:* a neural response to an abrupt stimulus such as a flash of light.

*Excitatory postsynaptic potential (EPSP):* a depolarizing graded potential that moves the cell membrane nearer to the threshold for initiating an action potential.

*Filter:* a device which removes or reduces certain parts of the input signal while allowing other parts of the signal to remain.

*Fistulated:* an animal with an artificial opening from an internal organ such as the stomach to the outside.

*Fluoroscope:* a device used to view objects exposed to X-rays.

*Fourier Analysis:* a method of breaking down a time series into the sine waves that make it up; a specific version of Fourier analysis often used by psychophysiologists is the Fast Fourier Transform or FFT.

*Frequency domain techniques:* techniques for analyzing data represented by different frequencies (or in the frequency domain).

*Gain:* amount of amplification.

*Galvanic Skin Response (GSR):* term replaced by electrodermal activity (EDA).

*Galvanometer:* a device used to determine the presence, strength, and direction of an electric current.

*Gamma band activity:* EEG activity in the 30 Hz to 70 Hz range assumed to be related to the brain's ability to integrate a variety of stimuli into a coherent whole.

*Ganglion:* a collection of nerve cells outside of the central nervous system.

*Gastroparesis:* an abnormal condition where the stomach fails to empty.

*Gaze Nystagmus:* see spontaneous nystagmus.

*Generator Potential:* the condition of a receptor after it has been excited and partially depolarized. If depolarization exceeds the axonal threshold, the generator potential produces a neural impulse.

*Graded Potential:* a change in potential across the cell membrane that is proportional to the amount of stimulation received. (See also excitatory postsynaptic potential and inhibitory postsynaptic potential.)

*Ground:* the connection (usually through a low-resistance conductor and the round prong on a three-pronged plug) of an electrical circuit or device with the earth.

*Habituation:* cessation of responding due to repeated presentation of the same stimulus.

*Heart period (HP) or Interbeat Interval (IBI):* the time between two consecutive heart beats; units usually in milliseconds.

*Heart rate (HR):* the rate of beating of the heart; units usually in beats/minute.

*Hering-Breuer Reflex:* inspiratory reflex evoked by stretch receptors in lung tissue that prevents overdistension of the lungs.

*High-pass Filter:* allows only frequencies above a certain frequency to pass.

*Homeostatic State:* steady-state internal environment providing the right temperature, nourishment, oxygen, and fluids for optimum functioning of all cells in a given region of the body.

*Hormone:* a chemical messenger which acts on receptors at relatively distant sites from its source and which reaches the receptor by way of the blood stream.

*Hyperpolarization:* enhancement of polarity; typically occurs when the inside of a neuron becomes more negatively charged relative to the outside and therefore less likely to generate an action potential.

*Impedance:* total resistance to current of an AC circuit; varies with the volume of a conductor and other factors.

*Impedance cardiography:* a non-invasive technique whereby a high frequency, low amplitude alternating current is passed through the chest to determine stroke volume, cardiac output, and systolic time intervals (such as pre-ejection period).

*Individual Response Stereotypy:* refers to the fact that individuals differ from one another in their pattern of bodily response to different situations; a given individual tends to show the greatest degree of activity in the same physiological system no matter what the situation.

*Inhibitory postsynaptic potential (IPSP):* a hyperpolarizing graded potential that moves the cell membrane further from the threshold for initiating an action potential.

*Inspiratory duty cycle (or inspiration fraction):* the inspiratory duration divided by the total duration of a respiratory cycle.

*Integrated Circuit (IC):* a multicomponent device (transistors, resistors, capacitors, etc.) in which the components have been miniaturized and designed for specific purposes.

*International 10–20 System:* a system which makes possible standardized placement of EEG electrodes on the scalp.

*Interstitial Fluid:* fluid found between the cells of the body; serves as a nutrient medium for the cells.

*Ion:* atom which has lost or gained an electron and is thereby capable of conducting electricity; a charged particle.

*Joint Interval Histogram:* method of presenting the results of frequency analysis of an EEG.

*Korotkoff Sounds:* used to determine blood pressure; the sounds are caused by turbulence in the blood as it spurts through the tiny arterial opening under the blood pressure cuff during each systole.

*Latency:* duration from stimulus presentation to response onset.

*Lateralized readiness potential (LRP):* A cortical measure of preparation for a motor response computed by subtracting the readiness potential of one hemisphere from that of the other.

*Law of Initial Values (LIV):* states that the initial state of a physiological system will limit the degree to which the system can change it's state; higher initial levels will limit further increases in function and lower initial levels will limit further decreases in function; this "law" is not always observed.

*Low-pass Filter:* allows only frequencies below a certain frequency to pass.

*Magnetic resonance imaging (MRI):* A system for measuring brain activity based on blood flow increases in active areas of the cortex. Hemoglobin which carries oxygen in the bloodstream has different magnetic properties before and after oxygen is absorbed. Magnetic fields are measured in MRI in relation to an external magnet.

*Magnetoencephalogram (MEG):* uses a SQUID (superconducting quantum interference device) to detect the small magnetic field gradients exiting and entering the surface of the head that are produced when neurons are active.

*Mastoid Process:* a nipple-shaped protrusion of the temporal bone located behind the ear.

*Mean Arterial Pressure (MAP):* the average blood pressure in the vascular system at the point where the measurement is taken; also diastolic blood pressure plus one-third the pulse pressure; units of millimeters of mercury (mmHg).

*Mean Inspiratory Flow:* the tidal volume divided by the duration of inspiration; units typically milliliters/second.

*Microsiemen:* the unit of conductance that has replaced micromho.

*Monopolar Recording:* a recording method involving placement of one or more electrodes at a site(s) where a relatively large amount of electrical activity is generated, and the other electrode (known as the reference electrode) at a site where electrical activity is minimal.

*Motor (or Endplate) Potential:* sudden depolarization across the motor endplate of the neuromuscular junction that typically initiates an action potential in the muscle.

*Motor Unit:* motor neuron and the muscle fibers it innervates.

*Myelin Sheath:* white, fatty substance that forms a sheath around the axons of some nerves.

*Myosin:* contractile protein in muscle fibers; functions in conjunction with actin.

*Nodes of Ranvier:* local constriction in the myelin sheath.

*Nonlinear dynamical analysis:* a broad theoretical approach that seeks to describe patterns in random appearing signal such as the EEG.

*Norepinephrine (also called Noradrenaline):* neurotransmitter at all sympathetic postganglionic synapses (except sweat glands); also acts as a hormone when released from the adrenal medulla.

*Notch Filter:* reduces only a small range of frequencies while allowing all others to pass undiminished (e.g., 60 Hz notch filter).

*Nystagmus Movement:* oscillatory movement of the eye.

*Off-Line Computer Usage:* use of a computer to analyze stored data; allows for analysis without regard to how events happened in real time, as opposed to on-line or real time usage.

*Ohm's Law:* the relationship between current, voltage and resistance in any electrical circuit and described by the equation, I (current) = V (voltage) ÷ R (resistance).

*On-Line:* the functioning of a computer which is working in the same time frame as the experiment it is controlling.

*Optokinetic Nystagmus:* oscillatory eye movements elicited by a moving pattern containing repeated patterns.

*Orienting Response:* a specific pattern of reactions which occurs in response to novel stimuli.

*Outlier:* a data point or observation that is extreme relative to the data from the rest of the sample.

*Pacemaker Cells (Pacesetter Potentials):* cells which originate the electrical impulse which produces contraction.

*Parasympathetic Nervous System (PNS):* craniosacral division of the autonomic nervous system; usually activation of this system induces effects opposite to those of the sympathetic nervous system.

*Peripheral Nervous System:* all neural material outside the brain and spinal cord.

*Positron emission tomography (PET):* radioactive system to measure variations in cerebral blood flow that are correlated with brain activity.

*Phasic (or Event-related) Activity:* a discrete response to a specific stimulus.

*Photoconductive Cell:* consists of a light source and a photoelectric cell which varies in electrical activity in proportion to the amount of light that hits the cell.

*Pilomotor Muscles:* those muscles that control elevation of body hair.

*Plethysmography:* the measurement of the size of a part of the body as a function of the volume it contains (typically volume of blood or air).

*Pneumograph:* a distensible air-filled tube, used for measuring respiration, that is placed around the subject's chest and connected to a pressure-sensitive device, an amplifier, and a computer or recorder.

*Polarization:* the difference in charge between the outside and inside of a membrane.

*Polygraph:* a device for recording two or more signals which are amplified and then written out on paper.

*Power Spectrum (or Spectral Density Plot):* a depiction of a physiological signal in the frequency domain that shows the component frequencies making up that signal.

*Preamplifier:* a device which conditions and amplifies input signals before they reach the power amplifier.

*Pre-ejection Period (PEP):* the time between the initiation of the electrical signal to the heart (usually the Q wave of the ECG) and the beginning of ejection of blood from the left ventricle; units are milliseconds.

*Pre-pulse Inhibition:* The act of presenting a less intense stimulus prior to the startle stimulus which decreases the startle response.

*Psychogalvanic Reflex (PGR):* an outdated term for skin conductance response.

*Pulse Pressure (PP):* the difference between the systolic blood pressure and the diastolic pressure; i.e., systolic blood pressure minus diastolic pressure; units of millimeters of mercury (mmHg).

*Pulse Volume:* a measure of the amplitude of individual pulses of blood in the vascular system.

*Pulse Wave Transit Time (PWTT):* time it takes for a pulse wave to travel from the heart to a distant location; related to blood pressure.

*Pupillography:* the measurement of the size of the pupil.

*Readiness Potential:* a slow negative potential, as recorded in an EEG, which precedes (by as much as 1.5 sec) and accompanies movement or other responses.

*Real Time:* (See On-Line).

*Receptor (or Generator) Potential:* a graded change in potential across the membrane after a receptor has been bound; if depolarization occurs and exceeds threshold, the receptor potential produces a neural impulse.

*Resistance:* a measure of the opposition that a conductor offers to the passage of current; it is the reciprocal of conductance.

*Respiratory Sinus Arrhythmia (RSA):* the rhythmic increases and decreases in heart rate produced by normal respiration; heart rate is increased during inspiration and decreased during expiration.

*Resting Potential:* the state of a neuron when it is conducive to transmitting a neural impulse specifically, when there is a difference in charge across its membrane. Also called the polarized state.

*Reticular Activating System (RAS):* reticular formation, thalamus, hypothalamus, and related structures which function to maintain appropriate states of arousal.

*Saccadic Eye Movement:* rapid jumping of the eyes from one fixation point to another, as during reading.

*Sampling Rate:* frequency with which sequential discrete samples of an analog physiological signal are recorded; units typically in Hz (samples/second).

*S-A Node: see* Sinoatrial Node.

*Schmitt Trigger:* a device which electronically checks for a certain voltage level and then signals a computer when it occurs.

*Sham feeding:* feeding that does not reach the stomach. In humans modified sham feeding is accomplished by having participants chew and then spit out the food; in lower animals surgery is used to remove food that has been swallowed from the gastrointestinal tract before it reaches the stomach.

*Signal Conditioner: See* Coupler.

*Signal-to-noise Ratio:* amount of signal (biopotential) in relation to other electrical activity (noise).

*Sinoatrial Node (S-A Node):* a small strip of electrically active muscle located in the upper part of the right atrium of the heart where the impulse that produces contraction of the heart begins.

*Skeletal Muscles:* those that move the trunk and limbs.

*Skin Conductance Level (SCL):* the reciprocal of the measure of how much resistance the skin of an organism in a state of rest or basal activity offers to passage of an electrical current (i.e., the reciprocal of skin resistance level); measured in mhos.

*Skin Conductance Response (SCR):* the reciprocal of the measure of how much resistance the skin of an organism that is responding to a particular stimulus offers to passage of an electrical current (i.e., the reciprocal of skin resistance response); measured in mhos.

*Skin Potential Level (SPL):* measure of electrical activity at the surface of the skin when the organism is in a state of rest or basal activity.

*Skin Potential Response (SPR):* measure of electrical activity at the surface of the skin when the organism is responding to a specific stimulus.

*Smooth Muscle:* unstriped muscle usually located in visceral walls and blood vessels.

*Smooth Pursuit Movement:* slow, apparently involuntary movements of the eyes which occur when a person is viewing a moving visual field.

*Somatic:* refers to the body.

*Somatic nervous system:* the portion of the nervous system controlling the skeletal muscles.

*Spectral Analysis:* a technique for determining the power of the frequencies present in a physiological record.

*Sphygmomanometer:* a device used to measure blood pressure, consisting of a pressure cuff connected to a vertical column containing mercury.

*Spirometry:* technique for directly measuring the volume of air inspired or expired during breathing.

*Spontaneous ANS Response:* a change in ANS activity that occurs in the absence of any known stimulus.

*Spontaneous Electroencephalogram:* continually occurring patterns of brain wave activity, as distinguished from event-related potentials.

*Spontaneous Nystagmus (Gaze Nystagmus):* oscillatory movements of the eye related to certain neurological disorders.

*Startle Response:* occurs to an intense stimulus with a sudden onset; characterized by a reflexive eyeblink, heart rate acceleration, and a rapid habituation.

*Stepwise Cross Correlation:* used, among other things, to determine time differences in similar EEG activity recorded from two sites.

*Stimulus-Response Specificity:* principle that specific stimulus situations bring about certain patterns of responding in most subjects, not just an increase or a decrease in a unidimensional activation continuum.

*Strain-Gauge Transducer:* sensing device that changes in electrical resistance as a function of the degree to which it is stretched; used to measure respiration, for example.

*Stretch receptors:* sensory receptors sensitive to the stretch or deformation of tissues.

*Striated Muscle:* see Skeletal Muscle.

*String Galvanometer:* early device used for recording the EKG.

*Sympathetic Nervous System (SNS):* thoracolumbar division of the autonomic nervous system; usually activation of this system induces effects opposite those of the parasympathetic nervous system.

*Sympathicotonic:* an individual who shows an unusually large response to drugs which stimulate the sympathetic nervous system.

*Symptom Specificity: See* Individual Response Stereotypy.

*Synapse:* the gap between two contiguous neurons along with the axon terminals of the presynaptic neuron and the receptive membrane of the postsynaptic neuron.

*Synaptic cleft:* the space or gap between contiguous neurons.

*Synaptic Functional Unit:* a group of cortical neurons sharing the same presynaptic input.

*Systolic Blood Pressure (SBP):* the maximal pressure in the vascular system at the point where the measurement is taken; systolic blood pressure occurs at the peak of the pressure pulse; units of millimeters of mercury (mmHg).

*Tachygastria:* an abnormally fast rate of incomplete gastric contractions often associated with delayed gastric emptying and reports of nausea.

*Telemetry:* a method for collecting psychophysiological data involving a transmitter (affixed to the subject) and receiver; eliminates need for direct connections between the subject and the recording equipment.

*Thermistor:* a device which changes electrical resistance in relation to changes in its temperature.

*Thermocouple:* a device which changes voltage in relation to changes in its temperature.

*Thermoresistive Transducer (Thermistor:* a device which changes in electrical resistance in relation to its temperature.

*Theta Activity:* refers to EEG activity in the 4–8 Hz range.

*Tidal volume:* The amount of air entering the lungs in a single breath; units typically in milliliters.

*Time Constant:* the amount of time required for a signal to return to 63 percent of its voltage.

*Time domain techniques:* techniques for analyzing data represented across time (or in the time domain).

*Tonic Level:* background or basal level of ANS or muscle activity.

*Torsional Eye Movements:* rotation movements around the line of gaze; smooth and compensatory.

*Transducer:* a device that changes one form of energy or activity into another.

*Vagotonic:* an individual who shows an unusually large response to drugs which stimulate the parasympathetic nervous system.

*Vasomotor Activity:* producing contraction or dilation in the walls of blood vessels.

*Vergence Eye Movements:* movement of the eyes in opposite directions so that objects moving toward or away from the eyes always appear as one object.

*Vestibular Nystagmus:* oscillatory eye movements elicited by head movement in which the semicircular canals are stimulated.

*Viscera:* internal organs of the body.

*Visual Evoked Response:* a predictable succession of brain wave forms and distribution observed after the subject is exposed to each of a series of flashes of light; of maximum amplitude over the occipital areas of the brain.

*Wavelet analysis:* a technique for determining frequency components of a signal. One advantage of this technique is its ability to work with short term signals.

# Index

dual process theory of habituation, 56
Duffy, E., 53

eccrine sweat glands, 209–10, 217, 222
ECG. *See* electrocardiography
EDA. *See* electrodermal activity
EEG. *See* electroencephalogram
efferent fiber, 17–19
efferent neuron, 15, 18
EGG. *See* electrogastrography
Einthoven, Willem, 9, 186
EKG. *See* electrocardiography
electricity
  of heart, 180–81
  safety in laboratory, 70–71
  of skin, 7–8
electric shock, 71–72
electrocardiography (EKG/ECG), 180–81
  arrhythmias, 182
  common problems, 189–90
  electrodes, 186–87
  recording procedure, 186–88
  typical recordings, 188
electrodermal activity (EDA), 206–19
  amplitude, 214–16, 219
  common problems, 213–14, 218–19
  electrodes, 211, 212, 218
  latency, 216, 219
  and lie detection, 252–53
  physiological basis, 209–11
  recovery time, 216–17
  skin conductance, 207–17
  skin potential, 217–19
  terminology, 207–9
  typical recordings, 213, 218
electrode(s), 36–39
  definition of, 36
  electrocardiography, 186–87
  electrodermal activity, 211, 212, 218
  electroencephalogram, 82–84
  electrogastrography, 164–65
  electromyography, 109–12, 116–17, 119–21
  electrooculography, 135–37
  and event-related potentials, 97

impedance and chemical stability, 36–37, 113
  paste, 39, 85
  polarization, 37
  potential or voltage produced by, 37
  and skin conductance, 211, 212
  skin preparation for, 39, 112–13
electroencephalogram (EEG), 79–91, 224
  alpha activity, 80, 224, 246
  analysis and quantification, 90–91
  Berger's early work, 9, 79–80
  and brain, 100–101, 249, 255
  common problems, 87–89
  electrodes, 82–84
  and event-related potentials, 96–98
  recording procedure, 82–85
  typical recordings, 86–87
  wavelet analysis, 236
electrogastrography (EGG), 157–74
  amplitude, 163–64, 166, 167
  cold pressor test, 168
  common problems, 170–71
  eating and sham feeding, 166–67
  electrodes, 164–65
  future directions, 174
  and gastric motor activity, 162–64
  and gastric myoelectric activity, 160–62
  and motion sickness, 169
  physiological basis, 158–64
  recording procedure, 164–66
  spectral analysis, 171–74
  typical recordings, 166–70
electromyography (EMG), 106–23
  analysis and quantification, 121–23
  common problems, 115–21
  electrodes, 109–12, 116–17, 119–21
  physiological basis, 108–9
  recording procedure, 109–13
  typical recordings, 114
electronic scanning, 129
electrooculography (EOG), 135–40
  analysis and quantification, 139–40

respiratory inductive
plethysmography, 149–50
respiratory sinus arrhythmia, 143,
145, 185
respiratory system, 142–55
physiological basis, 145–47
potential problems in recordings,
152–53
recording procedures, 147–52
respiration amplitude, 142, 154
respiration power spectrum, 232,
236–37
respiration rate, 142, 153
respiratory events, 154–55
response variables, 246
responsibility, 73–74
resting potential, 21, 24–25, 28–29
ribcage, 146, 147, 150

saccadic eye movement, 132, 133
safety, 70–72
saltatory conduction, 30
sampling rate, 44, 222–25
schizophrenia, 131
self-control, 250
self-inductance, 149
sensitization, 56
sensory systems, 15
signal-averaging procedures, 97–98
signal processing, 221–39
signal-to-noise ratio, 43
sine waves, 231, 234
size principle, 17
skeletal muscle. See striate muscle
skin
electrical properties of, 7–8
electrodermal activity, 206–19
preparation for electrodes, 39, 112–
13
resistance, 7–8
skin conductance, 207–17
conversion from resistance
readings, 214
recording procedure, 211–12
responses, 222
See also electrodermal activity
skin potential, 217–19
sleep, 87, 130–31, 247
slow potentials, 93–96, 101
smooth muscle, 28–29

smooth pursuit movements, 131,
132, 133
Society for Psychophysiological
Research, 5
sodium, 25
Sokolov, E. N., 56
somatic responses, 47
somatic system, 16–17
spectral analysis, 171–74
spectral density plot, 231
sphygmomanometer, 195–96
spinal cord, 16, 18, 20
spirometry, 147–48, 154
spontaneous electroencephalogram.
See electroencephalogram
spontaneous responses, 47–49
SQUID (superconducting quantum
interference device), 102
stability, 59
standards, 74
startle response, 58, 106–7
state variables, 247
Stern, John, 3
stimulus-response specificity, 6, 54,
65–66
stimulus/situational variables, 246–
47
strain gauge, 150–52
strain gauge plethysmography, 200–
201
strain gauge transducer, 40, 150
striate muscle, 26–28
string galvanometer, 9, 186
subject variables, 247–49
superconducting quantum
interference device. See SQUID
sweat glands, 209–11
sympathetic nervous system, 17–19,
22–23, 60
and autonomic control, 61–62
and blood flow, 179
and cardiac responding, 183–85
sympathicotonics, 60
synapse, 30–32, 97
synaptic cleft, 31
syncytia, 29
systolic blood pressure, 194–95

tachycardia, 181
Tallon-Baudry, Catherine, 80